Cell-Free Circulating DNA

Purification and Analysis Techniques

Cell-Free Circulating DNA

Purification and Analysis Techniques

Editors

Kristina Warton
University of New South Wales, Australia

Goli Samimi
National Cancer Institute, USA

World Scientific

NEW JERSEY · LONDON · SINGAPORE · BEIJING · SHANGHAI · HONG KONG · TAIPEI · CHENNAI · TOKYO

Published by

World Scientific Publishing Co. Pte. Ltd.

5 Toh Tuck Link, Singapore 596224

USA office: 27 Warren Street, Suite 401-402, Hackensack, NJ 07601

UK office: 57 Shelton Street, Covent Garden, London WC2H 9HE

British Library Cataloguing-in-Publication Data
A catalogue record for this book is available from the British Library.

ISBN 978-981-124-467-4 (hardcover)
ISBN 978-981-124-468-1 (ebook for institutions)
ISBN 978-981-124-469-8 (ebook for individuals)

For any available supplementary material, please visit
https://www.worldscientific.com/worldscibooks/10.1142/12494#t=suppl

Typeset by Stallion Press
Email: enquiries@stallionpress.com

Preface

Over the past decade a paradigm shift has occurred in the field of circulating diagnostics and personalized oncology that has been enabled by a dramatic expansion in high sensitivity technologies and instrumentation. This shift has its foundations in a series of discoveries that span more than a century and a half of clinical research. The initial observation of circulating tumour cells (CTCs) in the peripheral blood by the Australian physician Thomas Ashworth was published in 1869. The second fundamental discovery was the presence of small fragments of cell-free DNA (cfDNA) in blood by Mandel and Metais in 1948. Following on from this Leon (1977) and Stroun (1989) determined that a fraction of the cfDNA present in the blood of cancer patients was linked to their tumour. Together, these biological findings delivered the critical understanding that important genomic information is present in the peripheral blood and has potential diagnostic application.

Although the early implementation of both CTCs and cfDNA was focused on cancer prognostication and the detection of fetal DNA, it wasn't until 2010 when Pantel and Alix-Panabieres proposed the term liquid biopsy that its broad diagnostic utility as a minimally-invasive decision making tool was fully appreciated. The liquid biopsy concept quickly evolved to include any analyte present in different biological fluids that could be harnessed for diagnostic purposes. At the same time, the rise in the availability of highly sensitive detection instrumentation, including next generation sequencing and digital PCR (dPCR), has enhanced the ability to detect and interrogate these analytes. This has opened the way for liquid biopsies to be increasingly integrated into clinical diagnostic workflows alongside traditional invasive tissue biopsy. From a cancer perspective, the liquid biopsy of choice is circulating tumour DNA (ctDNA); it can be applied in different cancer scenarios including early detection, minimal residual disease, recurrence and treatment response monitoring, and can provide a representative cross-section of tumour heterogenicity.

The rapid advances in ctDNA technologies have resulted in pronouncements that we are now in the golden age of liquid biopsy research. However, there are still many biological, technical standardisation and other pre-analytical and clinical diagnostic issues (false negative/positive rates) that need to be addressed before the promise of liquid biopsy achieves its full potential. In particular, the issues surrounding technical variation and standardisation of workflows are important considerations for all in the field. The analytical validity of ctDNA assays has been mostly achieved, but there are still areas remaining that require attention such as clinical diagnostic assay validation and accreditation, along with the demonstration of assay clinical utility before implementation into routine clinical practice is possible. This book edited by Warton and Samimi is a timely and practical compilation of articles that will provide an important aid for researchers and clinicians wishing to utilize ctDNA for translational research, clinical trials and diagnostic purposes.

The first chapter focusing on the biology of cfDNA is a fundamental area of research interest. The understanding of cfDNA biology is important as new knowledge on cfDNA origin, shedding, fragmentation and dynamics can advance the development of new analytical approaches and potentially improve pre-analytical processing. The subsequent three chapters reinforce the need to be aware of critical pre-analytical factors, including sample type, as well as sample collection, processing and storage that may significantly affect the reproducibility and analytical accuracy of downstream assays. Quality assurance aspects involving internal and external controls, and reference materials are covered, as well as considerations for biobanking in the context of clinical trials. Pre-planning and careful attention to numerous logistical and sample variables, including extraction methods is required to ensure sufficient sample is available for biomarker evaluation and assay development and is clearly set out by the authors in these chapters. A detailed examination of factors influencing extraction performance and an extensive review of extraction methods and kits is provided in Chapter Four and should serve as a useful guide for choosing the most appropriate method or kit. Another pre-analytical factor that has been under-considered is blood DNases and their effects on cfDNA samples and is presented in Chapter Seven.

Knowing the intended analytical technique is important as it influences the extraction method chosen, for example targeting methylated cfDNA, mitochondrial cfDNA or total cfDNA. However, the final assay to be performed is not always known, especially for biobanked samples earmarked for future unspecified research, or due to the development of new analytical techniques. Chapters Five and Six consider the analytical phase of cfDNA liquid biopsies and focus on qPCR, dPCR and next generation sequencing. In addition, potential for PCR and sequencing biases exists and require careful consideration of sample preparation approaches.

Tailoring these techniques for the analysis of cfDNA and the critical factors involved is discussed in detail by the authors.

The final chapters reflect on circulating extracellular vesicles (EV) and exosomes in addition to the application of methylated DNA analysis. The authors summarise the origin and potential for these EV/exosome based biomarkers and describe some of the issues and challenges that still exist. The epigenetic analysis of circulating methylated DNA is highly topical and has generated great interest in the liquid biopsy community, especially cell-of-origin methylation pattern analysis. The technology is now available that allows for the extraction and analysis of small quantities of fragmented methylated DNA. However, its application requires a good understanding of methylated DNA biology and these aspects are clearly and concisely described by the authors.

The growth of liquid biopsy research involving both genetic and non-genetic molecular targets has resulted in important new insights and a critical understanding of circulating biomarkers and their diagnostic utility. This book makes an important contribution to the field and contains a wealth of up-to-date information on circulating DNA techniques and summarises the major advances that are essential for the implementation of liquid biopsies into routine clinical practice.

Kevin J Spring

Contents

Preface   v

List of Contributors   xi

**Chapter 1   Biology of Circulating DNA
                in Health and Disease**   1

Ahuva Odenheimer-Bergman, Havell Markus and
Muhammed Murtaza

**Chapter 2   Preanalytics and Quality Control
                of Different Substrates for Circulating
                DNA Studies**   21

Fay Betsou and Wim Ammerlaan

**Chapter 3   Considerations in Biobanking Blood
                Samples and Plasma Volume for
                Circulating DNA Studies**   47

Kate Mahon, Goli Samimi and Kristina Warton

Chapter 4 Maximizing Yield from Plasma Circulating DNA Extraction **63**

Florence Mauger and Jean-François Deleuze

Chapter 5 Optimal Design of PCR Assays for Circulating DNA **113**

Rikke F. Andersen

Chapter 6 Preparation of Next-Generation Sequencing Libraries for Sequencing Circulating DNA **139**

Katrin Heider, Florent Mouliere and Christopher G. Smith

Chapter 7 Blood Nucleases Affecting Circulating DNA in Serum and Plasma **175**

Gustavo Barra

Chapter 8 Isolating Circulating Exosomes as Biomarkers: Challenges and Opportunities **209**

Alexander Semaan and Anirban Maitra

Chapter 9 DNA Methylation Analysis of Circulating DNA Biomarkers **247**

Kristina Warton, Clare Stirzaker, Goli Samimi and Susan Clark

Index 279

List of Contributors

Ahuva Odenheimer-Bergman
Translational Genomics Research Institute, Phoenix, AZ, USA

Dr. Havell Markus
Penn State College of Medicine, Hershey, PA, USA

Prof. Muhammed Murtaza
Translational Genomics Research Institute, Phoenix, AZ; Department of Surgery and Center for Human Genomics and Precision Medicine, University of Wisconsin-Madison, Madison, WI, USA

Prof. Fay Betsou
Laboratoire National de Santé, Luxemburg

Wim Ammerlaan
Integrated Biobank of Luxemburg, Luxemburg

Dr. Kate Mahon
Chris O'Brien Lifehouse, Sydney, Australia

Dr. Goli Samimi
National Cancer Institute, Bethesda, MD, USA

Dr. Kristina Warton
University of New South Wales, Sydney, Australia

Dr. Florence Mauger
Université Paris-Saclay, CEA, Centre National de Recherche en Génomique Humaine, Evry, France

Dr. Jean-François Deleuze
Université Paris-Saclay, CEA, Centre National de Recherche en Génomique Humaine, Evry, France

Dr. Rikke F. Andersen
Lillebaelt Hospital, Vejle, Denmark

Dr. Katrin Heider
University of Cambridge, Cambridge, UK

Dr. Florent Mouliere
University of Cambridge, Cambridge, UK

Dr. Christopher G. Smith
University of Cambridge, Cambridge, UK

Dr. Gustavo Barra
Sabin Medicina Diagnóstica, Brasilia, Brazil

Dr. Alexander Semaan
MD Anderson Cancer Center, Houston, USA

Prof. Anirban Maitra
MD Anderson Cancer Center, Houston, USA

A/Prof. Clare Stirzaker

Garvan Institute of Medical Research and St. Vincent's Clinical School, Faculty of Medicine, UNSW, Sydney, Australia

Prof. Susan Clark

Garvan Institute of Medical Research and St. Vincent's Clinical School, Faculty of Medicine, UNSW, Sydney, Australia

Chapter 1

Biology of Circulating DNA in Health and Disease

Ahuva Odenheimer-Bergman,
Havell Markus and Muhammed Murtaza

Abstract

Circulating tumor DNA (ctDNA) analysis holds tremendous diagnostic value throughout cancer management. Potential applications of ctDNA analysis include minimally invasive tumor genotyping, monitoring treatment response, tracking subclonal evolution, detecting recurrence or minimal residual disease, and early detection. While some applications are already clinically available, numerous clinical studies are currently ongoing across cancer subtypes and disease stages and several groups are developing and adapting molecular analysis methods ideally suited for each application. While excitement about potential clinical value of ctDNA analysis has mounted, our understanding of the biology of circulating DNA has lagged. Mechanisms of circulating DNA release from cells, degradation, and clearance remain poorly understood. Recent studies have shown that leveraging insights into circulating DNA biology when developing biomarkers greatly improves accuracy and clinical relevance. In this chapter, we describe current understanding and

1

unanswered questions about the biology of circulating DNA, particularly highlighting areas with relevance to preanalytical and analytical techniques and methods for biomarker development.

Introduction

The presence of extracellular DNA fragments in serum was first described by Mandel and in 1948.[1] Hundreds of studies have since evaluated circulating DNA as biomarkers using increasingly sophisticated molecular analysis methods, across multiple diseases and physiological conditions. Initial studies compared total circulating cell-free DNA (cirDNA) levels in serum or plasma between healthy individuals and patients with acute illnesses (such myocardial infarction, stroke, infections, or trauma) or with chronic diseases (such as cancer or autoimmune diseases). While cirDNA levels are generally higher in patients, they can rarely differentiate adequately between healthy and diseased individuals due to overlapping distributions. Enabled by advances in molecular analysis and sequencing technologies, recent efforts have focused on measuring disease-specific cirDNA fragments. Noninvasive prenatal diagnostics (NIPD) is the first successful example of such efforts, focusing on fetal DNA in plasma from pregnant mothers. Since the first definitive report detecting the presence of chrY DNA fragments (specific to male fetuses) in maternal plasma published in 1997,[2] advances in this field have already led to clinically validated and commercially available screening tests for fetal aneuploidies and changed the diagnostic paradigm in prenatal testing.[3]

The field of circulating tumor DNA (ctDNA) analysis hopes to emulate the success in NIPD. While several aspects of circulating DNA biology learnt from prenatal testing are relevant, there are unique challenges and opportunities in patients with cancer.

ctDNA analysis relies on measuring cell-free DNA fragments that carry somatic genomic alterations specific to cancer cells.[4] These include single nucleotide variants, small insertions and deletions, rearrangement breakpoints, as well as cancer-specific DNA methylation changes. In addition, ctDNA analysis can also measure differences in cell-free DNA abundance across genomic loci, reflecting somatic copy number aberrations.

The presence of cancer-specific mutations in cirDNA was first reported in the 1970s[5] and its clinical relevance was demonstrated in 2004.[6] Recent technological advances in molecular analysis and DNA sequencing have enabled several potential diagnostic applications including noninvasive tumor genotyping,[7] treatment monitoring,[8] tracking clonal evolution in advanced cancer patients,[9,10] recurrence monitoring and minimal residual disease detection in early stage cancer patients,[11,12] as well as early detection of cancer in pre-symptomatic individuals.[13,14] Among these applications, noninvasive tumor genotyping for patients with metastatic cancers is furthest in its development and available for clinical testing from multiple commercial service providers today.

Cancer-specific mutations identified in ctDNA from plasma samples are generally concordant with similar analysis performed on tumor tissue samples from the same patients with metastatic cancer, except when affected by tumor heterogeneity.[15] However, cancer mutations identified in tumor tissue can often be missed in plasma samples, highlighting the challenge of detecting low levels of ctDNA in plasma and the need for high-sensitivity analytical methods. Ongoing efforts in this area are focused on establishing consensus criteria for analytical and clinical validity and evaluating the clinical utility of ctDNA-based genotyping. Several examples in the literature demonstrate the relevance of ctDNA analysis for other diagnostic scenarios, but these generally still require further technical/analytical improvements and definitive evaluation of clinical validity.[16]

While excitement regarding clinical applications of ctDNA analysis across cancer types and diagnostic scenarios has grown, new insights into cell-free DNA biology have been limited. Recent studies have demonstrated how biological characteristics of cirDNA can be leveraged to enable novel diagnostic applications for cancer patients. For example, genomic positioning of cell-free DNA fragments in plasma was recently shown to reflect dynamic nucleosome positioning in the cells of origin, with nucleosome binding postulated to protect the DNA from digestion by plasma nucleases. This observation led to two novel potential applications in metastatic cancer patients, where ctDNA levels in plasma are often very high. First, it enabled inference of histological tumor cell type, with potential relevance for cancer patients with unknown primary tumor sites.[17] Second, with deeper sequencing and in a fraction of patients with the highest ctDNA levels, differential plasma DNA abundance at and around the transcription start sites enabled inference of gene expression in the tumor cells.[18] Another example of a biological insight enabling better diagnostics is observation of differences in ctDNA fragment size. Several studies have shown that while most plasma DNA fragments are mono-nucleosomal in size (~167 bp), fetal and tumor-derived DNA fragments tend to be shorter, potentially lacking nucleosome linker DNA regions due to differences in mechanisms of DNA degradation and release. Recent efforts are now relying on size selection of cell-free DNA fragments to enrich for tumor signal, either during sequencing library preparation or using informatics tools.[19]

To enable further such advances, in this chapter, we summarize current understanding and unanswered questions in circulating cell-free DNA biology, with a specific focus on areas relevant to diagnostic development.

Total Circulating Cell-Free DNA Concentration

Several studies have evaluated the diagnostic value of total cirDNA levels across disease types. Although significantly higher levels are often observed when comparing cancer patients with healthy volunteers, overlapping observations of total cirDNA levels between the two groups limit their diagnostic accuracy, at least in univariate analysis.[20] In addition, total cirDNA levels vary between individuals and are affected by physiological differences such as body mass index as well as disease states such as autoimmune and rheumatic disorders.[21,22] They are also affected by transient physiological conditions such as exercise or fasting. The effects of diet, food and fluid intake or fasting, physical activity, and time of the day (circadian rhythm) on total cirDNA and tumor-specific ctDNA remain poorly understood. For example, several studies have found exercise increases total cirDNA concentrations in healthy volunteers.[23–29] However, the source of the additional cirDNA released during exercise is unclear, and it is not known whether exercise or physical stress will transiently dilute tumor-specific mutation levels in cancer patients. Total cirDNA levels are also affected heavily by preanalytical factors such as delays between venipuncture and processing of blood samples, and differences between blood collection protocols and DNA extraction protocols.[30] Delays in blood processing or inappropriate blood collection protocols can lead to lysis of peripheral blood cells, leading to artifactual increases in total cirDNA. These unanswered questions further limit the utility of total cirDNA levels for cancer diagnostics.

cirDNA levels do not appear to be influenced by circadian rhythm; however, the data available is limited. In healthy volunteers, a comparison of total cirDNA levels in plasma samples obtained at different times of the day showed no significant difference.[31,32] In cancer patients, one recent study evaluated multiple plasma samples obtained from nine colorectal cancer patients at four different times of the day and suggested total cirDNA levels were lowest and tumor-specific ctDNA was most detectable at mid-night.[33] Based on these preliminary results, they inferred that daytime activity could potentially dilute tumor-derived DNA levels in circulation and an early morning sample may be most informative. Another study compared histone modifications in cirDNA between different times of blood collection and found no significant differences in 5mC or H3K9me3 histone modification levels.[34] Despite limitations, it is conceivable that total cirDNA levels may add value as part of multiparametric assessments, where total cirDNA levels are interpreted together with other variables such as tumor-specific ctDNA levels, fragmentation patterns, and size distributions.[35]

Total cirDNA levels also determine the amount of DNA available for analysis from a clinically obtainable volume of blood, a key variable that affects clinical assay sensitivity, accuracy, and precision. Despite several recent advances in detection of low abundance mutations using next-generation sequencing or digital PCR, actual sensitivity is often limited by low total cirDNA amounts available from patient samples and by loss of analyte due to technical inefficiencies. In healthy volunteers with no known cancers, total cirDNA concentration is typically 5–7 ng/mL of plasma (equivalent to 1500–2100 haploid genome copies or hGCs).[30] A 10 mL blood sample typically yields about 4 mL plasma, resulting in ~6000–8400 hGCs. Due to sampling variation, any molecular assay is expected to have limited sensitivity for individual mutations at <0.1% AF in 10 mL blood samples (<6–8 mutated DNA fragments available on average for detection for each mutation). Total cirDNA concentrations are expected to be similar in pre-symptomatic cancer patients (a screening or early detection population) or in localized cancer patients.[11,12] In contrast, plasma samples from metastatic cancer patients have higher total cirDNA concentrations and yield more analyte, circumventing concerns for sampling errors.[20]

Clinical Tumor Characteristics Affecting Circulating Tumor DNA Levels

ctDNA levels can be affected by biology of the tumor or clinical variables such as ongoing treatments. Differences in tumor doubling time, number of proliferating cells, and level of tumor loss can lead to different ctDNA levels across cancer types. For example, in one study, colorectal cancer was shown to have a doubling time of 90 days, cell loss factor of 96%, and level of cell proliferation of 15%, and patients with colorectal cancer have some of the highest levels of ctDNA.[15,36] In contrast, a different study showed thyroid cancer has a tumor doubling time of 212 days and ctDNA levels observed for thyroid cancer are typically much lower.[37,38] Within each tumor type, several studies have reported association of ctDNA levels with mitotic rate or Ki67 levels[39,40] as well as tumor vascularity and hypoxia.[41–43]

In recent studies of lung cancer, ctDNA levels have been correlated with tumor volume although such data are limited across most tumor types.[44] In addition, whether a linear correlation holds when tumor volumes are extremely low and undetectable on imaging is unclear. For example, a linear model of ctDNA levels prior to treatment with tumor volumes suggested ctDNA levels would be below limit of detection post-operatively using the same assay in one study.[39] However, ctDNA was detected in several cases with residual disease, suggesting that the model may not hold across tumor volumes or throughout stages of treatment and response. A potential explanation for a higher rate of ctDNA shedding from residual disease may be a more aggressive, growth phenotype in the systemic residual tumor upon resection of the primary site. Recent studies identify minimum tumor volumes where ctDNA is detectable, but these calculations are bound to be tumor-type specific and affected by the limit of detection for assays used.[45]

Tumor-derived ctDNA levels can be affected acutely due to treatment-related events. For example, ctDNA levels tend to spike within hours of surgical manipulation of the tumor or infusion of chemotherapy.[46,47] While a relationship with intravenously infused cytotoxic chemotherapy has been observed, how oral molecularly targeted agents or immune checkpoint inhibitors affect ctDNA levels acutely is not clear. In some studies, acute increases in tumor-specific ctDNA have been useful as markers of treatment response.[48,49]

Half-Life and ctDNA Clearance

Fetal DNA is cleared from maternal plasma using a two-phased clearance mechanism, which begins with a rapid clearance in the first 2-hr postpartum, and then a second slower phase, which takes up to 2 days postpartum to clear the remaining fetal DNA from maternal plasma.[50] Tumor-derived DNA has been observed to have a similar half-life of 114 min, observed in colorectal cancer patients after surgical resection.[6,47] Experimental studies evaluating the half-life of cirDNA have made similar observations. One group studied clearance of mono-nucleosomes with radiolabeled histones injected intravenously into mice and found that within 10 min, 70%–85% of the signal was detected in the liver and <1% found in the kidneys.[29,51]

To be finally cleared from the body, cirDNA degradation products are likely excreted in urine. However, mononucleosomes are unlikely to filter into urine through the glomeruli (90-kDa-sized mononucleosomes and a maximum size cutoff of 70 kDa). The negative charge of DNA likely lowers the permeability further. Although several groups have suggested observing cell-free DNA fragments of ~150 bp size in urine, whether such DNA is trans-renal or locally shed by the uro-epithelium is unclear and a mechanism that could facilitate filtration of mono-nucleosomes into urine is unknown. Other groups have observed much shorter DNA fragments in urine, suggesting further degradation of cirDNA prior to filtration and within the genitourinary tract.[50,52,53]

The ends of cirDNA fragments in plasma and urine reveal distinct but conserved sequence motifs across multiple studies, suggesting the role of distinct nucleases in DNA digestion in plasma and in urine.[53–55] Recent studies have shown that DNAse1-like3 is likely responsible for degrading chromatin in plasma while DNAse1 is more active in urine and acts on DNA not bound to nucleosomes. The sequence motifs on plasma DNA fragments show a preference for cytosine at the fragment ends, while those on urine DNA fragments show a preference for thymine.[53] These observations are consistent with the sequence motifs related to corresponding nucleases in plasma and urine.[56,57]

Circulating DNA Fragment Size and Positioning

Circulating DNA in plasma is predominantly fragmented to ~167 bp, corresponding to DNA length wrapped in mono-nucleosomes. Additional modal sizes are observed consistent with di-nucleosomes and tri-nucleosomes. In addition, the size distribution shows a 10 bp step pattern, suggesting enzymatic degradation.[58] These observations suggest cirDNA is shed during cell turnover by apoptosis, although alternative mechanisms for enzymatic degradation cannot be ruled out, such as secondary digestion of longer DNA fragments shed by necrosis by enzymes in the bloodstream, or release of fragmented DNA by phagocytes that engulf and digest dying cells.[6,59–61] Longer DNA fragments are observed in some blood samples, but it is generally assumed that these are contributed by lysis of cells in the bloodstream, either in vivo or during venipuncture and sample processing. Delays in and differences in preanalytical sample processing have been shown to increase fraction of longer DNA fragments in plasma samples and to lower measures of tumor-derived ctDNA.[30] In some patients with metastatic cancers with high tumor burden and necrotic tumors, it is likely that longer fragments are contributed by necrotic tumor cells.[62]

Assaying short fragments is a key consideration during circulating DNA analysis. Conventional DNA extraction approaches often prioritize intact over "degraded" DNA and this results in lost yield. Newer cirDNA-focused extraction methods can overcome this limitation. Similarly, any negative selection of shorter fragments downstream (e.g., during sequencing library preparation and cleanup) can lower effective yield. Due to ongoing degradation, sequencing library preparation that can capture single-stranded DNA has been shown to capture a larger fraction of cell-free DNA fragments shorter than 100 bp.[63] Short fragment size also limits the size of amplicons designed for target-specific PCR analysis (digital PCR or amplicon sequencing). Assuming cirDNA is fragmented randomly, the maximum fraction of DNA fragments captured by both PCR primers decreases with increasing amplicon size, predictable using the exponential distribution. For example, a 120-bp amplicon will capture ~45% of 150-bp DNA fragments, while a 71-bp amplicon will capture ~62% of ~150-bp DNA fragments.[30]

Recent studies have shown cirDNA fragmentation is not completely random and is consistent with protection from complete degradation by nucleosomes.[53,64] Using whole genome sequencing, studies found relative levels and periodicity in cirDNA abundance across genomic loci were consistent with micrococcal nuclease digestion, which cleaves DNA at inter-nucleosomal sites and has traditionally been used to map nucleosome positioning.[65] Actively transcribed genes have a nucleosome-depleted region at transcription start sites and in relative sequencing coverage in cirDNA at these genomic loci is correlated with gene expression in tissues that contribute cirDNA. In patients with advanced metastatic cancers where tumor-derived ctDNA fractions are high, sequencing coverage and fragment size at transcription start sites and known transcription factor-binding loci can be leveraged to identify primary tumor cell types and infer gene expression.[17,18,66] To maximize analytical yield and potentially enrich tumor-derived signal, design of PCR assays can be further informed by the nonrandom fragmentation of cirDNA. However, due to differences expected between contributing cell types, dynamic changes in nucleosome positioning, and inability to predict nucleosome positioning precisely for most genomic loci, no published ctDNA studies have leveraged nonrandom positioning to aid PCR assay design so far.

Several studies have observed that circulating DNA fragments shed by fetal cells or tumor cells tend to be shorter than maternal cells or healthy wild-type cells. In prenatal diagnostics studies, fetal-specific DNA has been found to have modal size of ~147 bp, about 20 bp shorter than maternal-specific DNA ~166 bp, and the relative fraction of these sizes could be used to infer fetal

DNA fraction in circulation.[58,67] A follow-up study demonstrated that cirDNA has preferential end sites (PES), genomic positions where fragments are more likely to be cleaved, associated with long and short fragments.[68] Using this set of long and short PES, it was shown that maternal cirDNA is more likely to be cleaved at long PES, and fetal cirDNA is more likely to be cleaved at short PES. Long PES associated with maternal DNA tend to fall in the linker region, while short PES associated with fetal DNA tend to fall closer to or within the nucleosome core. This observation suggests fetal DNA may be more accessible to nuclease cleavage than maternal DNA, perhaps due to more active transcription across the genome in rapidly proliferating cells. Selecting fragments to analyze based on the PES enabled a 90-fold enhancement in the resolution of the fetal genome.[69]

Similarly, relative shortening of circulating DNA has also been observed in tumor-derived DNA from plasma[70] and cerebro-spinal fluid,[71] and selection of shorter fragments before or after sequencing library preparation has been leveraged to enrich tumor signal.[19,72] Using in silico size selection, Jiang *et al.* showed a significant positive correlation between the proportion of fragments less than 150 bp and tumor DNA concentration in plasma of patients with hepatocellular carcinoma, while fragments between 150 and 180 bp showed no correlation.[70] Mouliere *et al.* selected fragments between 90 and 150 bp in plasma samples of patients with various cancer types and achieved a median 2-fold enrichment of ctDNA. Through size selection, they were also able to identify clinically relevant/actionable somatic mutations and copy number alteration events that were otherwise not observed.[19]

Cell-type-specific DNA organization and differences in processes underlying cell death can result in cirDNA with cell-type-specific nonrandom fragmentation signatures.[53] Chandrananda *et al.* described that cirDNA fragmentation in healthy plasma samples is not random as the sequences of first and last 10 bp of cirDNA fragments show a conserved pattern for nucleotide preference.[54] Chen *et al.* followed this observation and used the nucleotide motif present in the first and last 10 bp of fragments to build a machine learning classifier to distinguish cirDNA from plasma and urine, and samples from formalin-fixed paraffin embedded (FFPE) tumor DNA samples.[55] Although they did not find a conserved fragmentation pattern in cirDNA from cerebrospinal fluid, this could be due to a limited sample set or different processing methods. The study further showed that these fragmentation patterns are similar in every fragment size (long or short), thus suggesting short fragments present in circulation are not due to degradation of long fragments. Findings of these studies suggest cirDNA carries important structural and functional information that could potentially be used to improve bioinformatics algorithms to distinguish ctDNA among wild-type cirDNA based on molecular features in addition to fragment sizes.

It is unclear how much of the cirDNA in circulation is enclosed within membrane-bound vesicles or bound to cell surface.[73] Extracellular vesicles have been shown to contain multiple cellular components including proteins, microRNAs and messenger RNAs, as well as single- and double-stranded DNA.[74] In cancer patients, exosomes derived from tumors may carry double-stranded tumor-derived and mutated DNA.[75,76] This suggests selection of vesicles using membrane and cell-surface markers may enrich tumor-derived ctDNA signal, above background noise in molecular assays. However, any such gains in tumor fraction will have to be balanced against loss of material associated with enrichment strategies.[74,76,77]

Summary

Analysis of cell-free DNA has already transformed diagnostics in multiple areas of medicine, without much initial regard to biological determinants of cirDNA in health and disease. However, diagnostic development has arrived at stiff limits of detection for methods based on single nucleotide variants and polymorphisms that can no longer be overcome with greater depth of sequencing while analyzing feasible volumes of blood. This has spurned rapid progress into analysis of biological features of cirDNA that could be leveraged to improve diagnostic performance, making it the current frontier in this field. There are several unanswered questions that remain in cell-free DNA biology, which could have profound impacts on the choices and accuracy of preanalytical and analytical techniques used for cell-free DNA analysis.

References

1. Mandel P, Metais P. (1948) Les acides nucléiques du plasma sanguin chez l'homme. *C R Seances Soc Biol Fil* **142**: 241–243.
2. Lo YM, Corbetta N, Chamberlain PF, *et al.* (1997) Presence of fetal DNA in maternal plasma and serum. *Lancet* **350**: 485–487.
3. Wong FC, Lo YM. (2016) Prenatal diagnosis innovation: Genome sequencing of maternal plasma. *Annu Rev Med* **67**: 419–432.
4. Wan JC, Massie C, Garcia-Corbacho J, *et al.* (2017). Liquid biopsies come of age: Towards implementation of circulating tumour DNA. *Nat Rev Cancer* **17**: 223–238.
5. Leon S, Shapiro B, Sklaroff D, Yaros M. (1977) Free DNA in the serum of cancer patients and the effect of therapy. *Cancer Res* **37**: 646–650.
6. Diehl F, Li M, Dressman D, *et al.* (2005) Detection and quantification of mutations in the plasma of patients with colorectal tumors. *Proc Natl Acad Sci USA* **102**: 16368–16373.
7. Forshew T, Murtaza M, Parkinson C, *et al.* (2012) Noninvasive identification and monitoring of cancer mutations by targeted deep sequencing of plasma DNA. *Sci Transl Med* **4**: 136ra68–ra68.

8. Dawson SJ, Tsui DW, Murtaza M, *et al.* (2013) Analysis of circulating tumor DNA to monitor metastatic breast cancer. *N Engl J Med* **368**: 1199–1209.

9. Murtaza M, Dawson SJ, Pogrebniak K, *et al.* (2015) Multifocal clonal evolution characterized using circulating tumour DNA in a case of metastatic breast cancer. *Nat Commun* **6**: 8760.

10. Murtaza M, Dawson SJ, Tsui DW, *et al.* (2013) Non-invasive analysis of acquired resistance to cancer therapy by sequencing of plasma DNA. *Nature* **497**.

11. McDonald BR, Contente-Cuomo T, Sammut SJ, *et al.* (2019) Personalized circulating tumor DNA analysis to detect residual disease after neoadjuvant therapy in breast cancer. *Sci Transl Med* **11**: eaax7392.

12. McDonald BR, Contente-Cuomo T, Sammut S-J, *et al.* (2018) Detection of residual disease after neoadjuvant therapy in breast cancer using personalized circulating tumor DNA analysis. *bioRxiv*.

13. Phallen J, Sausen M, Adleff V, *et al.* (2017) Direct detection of early-stage cancers using circulating tumor DNA. *Sci Transl Med* **9**: eaan2415.

14. Cohen JD, Li L, Wang Y, *et al.* (2018) Detection and localization of surgically resectable cancers with a multi-analyte blood test. *Science* eaar3247.

15. Bettegowda C, Sausen M, Leary RJ, *et al.* (2014) Detection of circulating tumor DNA in early- and late-stage human malignancies. *Sci Transl Med* **6**: 224ra24.

16. Merker JD, Oxnard GR, Compton C, *et al.* (2018) Circulating tumor DNA analysis in patients with cancer: American Society of Clinical Oncology and College of American Pathologists joint review. *Arch Pathol Lab Med* **142**: 1242–1253.

17. Snyder MW, Kircher M, Hill AJ, *et al.* (2016) Cell-free DNA comprises an in vivo nucleosome footprint that informs its tissues-of-origin. *Cell* **164**: 57–68.

18. Ulz P, Thallinger GG, Auer M, *et al.* (2016) Inferring expressed genes by whole-genome sequencing of plasma DNA. *Nat Genet* **48**: 1273–1278.

19. Mouliere F, Chandrananda D, Piskorz AM, *et al.* (2018) Enhanced detection of circulating tumor DNA by fragment size analysis. *Sci Transl Med* **10**.

20. Farooq M, Egan JB, McDonald B, *et al.* (2018) Detection of copy number aberrations in cholangiocarcinoma using shallow whole genome sequencing of plasma DNA. *Am Soc Clin Oncol* **(36)4**, Abstract 293.

21. Duvvuri B, Lood C. (2019) Cell-free DNA as a biomarker in autoimmune rheumatic diseases. *Front Immunol* **10**: 502.

22. Vora NL, Johnson KL, Basu S, *et al.* (2012) A multifactorial relationship exists between total circulating cell-free DNA levels and maternal BMI. *Prenat Diagn* **32**: 912–914.

23. Hummel EM, Hessas E, Muller S, *et al.* (2018) Cell-free DNA release under psychosocial and physical stress conditions. *Transl Psychiatry* **8**: 236.

24. Tug S, Helmig S, Deichmann ER, *et al.* (2015) Exercise-induced increases in cell free DNA in human plasma originate predominantly from cells of the haematopoietic lineage. *Exerc Immunol Rev* **21**: 164–173.

25. Fruhbeis C, Helmig S, Tug S, *et al.* (2015) Physical exercise induces rapid release of small extracellular vesicles into the circulation. *J Extracell Vesicles* **4**: 28239.

26. Breitbach S, Tug S, Simon P. (2012) Circulating cell-free DNA: An up-coming molecular marker in exercise physiology. *Sports Med* **42**: 565–586.

27. Velders M, Treff G, Machus K, *et al.* (2014) Exercise is a potent stimulus for enhancing circulating DNase activity. *Clin Biochem* **47**: 471–474.

28. Chevion S, Moran DS, Heled Y, *et al.* (2003) Plasma antioxidant status and cell injury after severe physical exercise. *Proc Natl Acad Sci USA* **100**: 5119–5123.

29. Pokrywka A, Zembron-Lacny A, Baldy-Chudzik K, *et al.* (2015) The influence of hypoxic physical activity on cfDNA as a new marker of vascular inflammation. *Arch Med Sci* **11**: 1156–1163.

30. Markus H, Contente-Cuomo T, Farooq M, *et al.* (2018) Evaluation of pre-analytical factors affecting plasma DNA analysis. *Sci Rep* **8**: 7375.

31. Korabecna M, Horinek A, Bila N, Opatrna S. (2011) Circadian rhythmicity and clearance of cell-free DNA in human plasma. In *Circulating Nucleic Acids in Plasma and Serum.* Springer Netherlands, Dordrecht, pp. 195–198.

32. Marie Korabecna AH, Nikola B, Sylvie O. (2010) Circadian rhythmicity and clearance of cell-free DNA in human plasma. *Circulating Nucleic Acids in Plasma and Serum.*

33. Toth K, Patai AV, Kalmar A, *et al.* (2017) Circadian rhythm of methylated septin 9, cell-free DNA amount and tumor markers in colorectal cancer patients. *Pathol Oncol Res* **23**: 699–706.

34. Rasmussen L, Herzog M, Romer E, *et al.* (2016) Pre-analytical variables of circulating cell-free nucleosomes containing 5-methylcytosine DNA or histone modification H3K9Me3. *Scand J Clin Lab Invest* **76**: 448–453.

35. Mouliere F, El Messaoudi S, Pang D, *et al.* (2014) Multi-marker analysis of circulating cell-free DNA toward personalized medicine for colorectal cancer. *Mol Oncol* **8**: 927–941.

36. Ota DM, Drewinko B. (1985) Growth kinetics of human colorectal carcinoma. *Cancer Res* **45**: 2128–2131.

37. Thierry AR, El Messaoudi S, Gahan PB, *et al.* (2016) Origins, structures, and functions of circulating DNA in oncology. *Cancer Metastasis Rev* **35**: 347–376.

38. Rossing RM, Jentzen W, Nagarajah J, *et al.* (2016) Serum thyroglobulin doubling time in progressive thyroid cancer. *Thyroid* **26**: 1712–1718.

39. Abbosh C, Birkbak NJ, Wilson GA, *et al.* (2017) Phylogenetic ctDNA analysis depicts early-stage lung cancer evolution. *Nature* **545**: 446–451.

40. Riva F, Bidard FC, Houy A, *et al.* (2017) Patient-specific circulating tumor DNA detection during neoadjuvant chemotherapy in triple-negative breast cancer. *Clin Chem* **63**: 691–699.

41. Weidner N. (2002) New paradigm for vessel intravasation by tumor cells. *Am J Pathol* **160**: 1937–1939.

42. Lee SY, Chao-Nan Q, Seng OA, *et al.* (2012) Changes in specialized blood vessels in lymph nodes and their role in cancer metastasis. *J Transl Med* **10**: 206.

43. Qian CN, Tan MH, Yang JP, Cao Y. (2016) Revisiting tumor angiogenesis: Vessel co-option, vessel remodeling, and cancer cell-derived vasculature formation. *Chin J Cancer* **35**: 10.

44. Avanzini S, Kurtz DM, Chabon JJ, *et al.* (2020) A mathematical model of ctDNA shedding predicts tumor detection size. *Sci Adv.* 6(50):eabc4308.

45. Chabon JJ, Hamilton EG, Kurtz DM, *et al.* (2020) Integrating genomic features for non-invasive early lung cancer detection. *Nature* **580**: 245–251.

46. Siravegna G, Bardelli A. (2014) Genotyping cell-free tumor DNA in the blood to detect residual disease and drug resistance. *Genome Biol* **15**: 449.

47. Diehl F, Schmidt K, Choti MA, *et al.* (2008) Circulating mutant DNA to assess tumor dynamics. *Nat Med* **14**: 985–990.

48. Husain H, Melnikova VO, Kosco K, *et al.* (2017) Monitoring daily dynamics of early tumor response to targeted therapy by detecting circulating tumor DNA in urine. *Clin Cancer Res* **23**: 4716–4723.

49. Xi L, Pham TH, Payabyab EC, *et al.* (2016) Circulating tumor DNA as an early indicator of response to T-cell transfer immunotherapy in metastatic melanoma. *Clin Cancer Res* **22**: 5480–5486.

50. Lo YM, Zhang J, Leung TN, *et al.* (1999) Rapid clearance of fetal DNA from maternal plasma. *Am J Hum Genet* **64**: 218–224.

51. Gauthier VJ, Tyler LN, Mannik M. (1996) Blood clearance kinetics and liver uptake of mononucleosomes in mice. *J Immunol* **156**: 1151–1156.

52. Cheng THT, Jiang P, Tam JCW, *et al.* (2017) Genomewide bisulfite sequencing reveals the origin and time-dependent fragmentation of urinary cfDNA. *Clin Biochem* **50**: 496–501.

53. Markus H, Zhao J, Contente-Cuomo T, *et al.* (2021) Analysis of recurrently protected genomic regions in cell-free DNA found in urine. *Sci Transl Med* **13**.

54. Chandrananda D, Thorne NP, Bahlo M. (2015) High-resolution characterization of sequence signatures due to non-random cleavage of cell-free DNA. *BMC Med Genomics* **8**: 29.

55. Chen S, Liu M, Zhang X, *et al.* (2017) A study of cell-free DNA fragmentation pattern and its application in DNA sample type classification. *IEEE/ACM Trans Comput Biol Bioinform.*

56. Han DSC, Ni M, Chan RWY, *et al.* (2020) The biology of cell-free DNA fragmentation and the roles of DNASE1, DNASE1L3, and DFFB. *Am J Hum Genet* **106**: 202–214.

57. Serpas L, Chan RWY, Jiang P, *et al.* (2019) Dnase1l3 deletion causes aberrations in length and end-motif frequencies in plasma DNA. *Proc Natl Acad Sci USA* **116**: 641–649.

58. Lo YM, Chan KC, Sun H, *et al.* (2010) Maternal plasma DNA sequencing reveals the genome-wide genetic and mutational profile of the fetus. *Sci Transl Med* **2**: 61ra91.

59. Mouliere F, Robert B, Arnau Peyrotte E, *et al.* (2011) High fragmentation characterizes tumour-derived circulating DNA. *PLoS One* **6**: e23418.

60. Tamkovich SN, Cherepanova AV, Kolesnikova EV, *et al.* (2006) Circulating DNA and DNase activity in human blood. *Ann N Y Acad Sci* **1075**: 191–196.

61. Rostami A, Lambie M, Yu CW, *et al.* (2020) Senescence, necrosis, and apoptosis govern circulating cell-free DNA release kinetics. *Cell Rep* **31**: 107830.

62. Ungerer V, Bronkhorst AJ, Van den Ackerveken P, *et al.* (2021) Serial profiling of cell-free DNA and nucleosome histone modifications in cell cultures. *Sci Rep* **11**: 9460.

63. Burnham P, Kim MS, Agbor-Enoh S, *et al.* (2016) Single-stranded DNA library preparation uncovers the origin and diversity of ultrashort cell-free DNA in plasma. *Sci Rep* **6**: 27859.

64. Murtaza M, Caldas C. (2016) Nucleosome mapping in plasma DNA predicts cancer gene expression. *Nat Genet* **48**: 1105–1106.

65. Schones DE, Cui K, Cuddapah S, *et al.* (2008) Dynamic regulation of nucleosome positioning in the human genome. *Cell* **132**: 887–898.

66. Ulz P, Perakis S, Zhou Q, *et al.* (2019) Inference of transcription factor binding from cell-free DNA enables tumor subtype prediction and early detection. *Nat Commun* **10**: 4666.

67. Yu SC, Chan KC, Zheng YW, *et al.* (2014) Size-based molecular diagnostics using plasma DNA for noninvasive prenatal testing. *Proc Natl Acad Sci USA* **111**: 8583–8588.

68. Chan KC, Jiang P, Sun K, *et al.* (2016) Second generation noninvasive fetal genome analysis reveals de novo mutations, single-base parental inheritance, and preferred DNA ends. *Proc Natl Acad Sci USA* **113**: E8159–E8168.

69. Sun K, Jiang P, Wong AIC, *et al.* (2018) Size-tagged preferred ends in maternal plasma DNA shed light on the production mechanism and show utility in noninvasive prenatal testing. *Proc Natl Acad Sci USA* **115**: E5106–E5114.

70. Jiang P, Chan CW, Chan KC, *et al.* (2015) Lengthening and shortening of plasma DNA in hepatocellular carcinoma patients. *Proc Natl Acad Sci USA* **112**: E1317–E1325.

71. Mouliere F, Mair R, Chandrananda D, *et al.* (2018) Detection of cell-free DNA fragmentation and copy number alterations in cerebrospinal fluid from glioma patients. *EMBO Mol Med* **10**: e9323.

72. Underhill HR, Kitzman JO, Hellwig S, *et al.* (2016) Fragment length of circulating tumor DNA. *PLoS Genet* **12**: e1006162.

73. Bryzgunova OE, Tamkovich SN, Cherepanova AV, *et al.* (2015) Redistribution of free- and cell-surface-bound DNA in blood of benign and malignant prostate tumor patients. *Acta Naturae* **7**: 115–118.

74. Bang C, Thum T. (2012) Exosomes: New players in cell-cell communication. *Int J Biochem Cell Biol* **44**: 2060–2064.

75. Melo SA, Luecke LB, Kahlert C, *et al.* Glypican-1 identifies cancer exosomes and detects early pancreatic cancer. *Nature* **523**: 177–182.

76. Thakur BK, Zhang H, Becker A, *et al.* (2014) Double-stranded DNA in exosomes: A novel biomarker in cancer detection. *Cell Res* **24**: 766–769.

77. van der Pol E, Boing AN, Harrison P, *et al.* (2012) Classification, functions, and clinical relevance of extracellular vesicles. *Pharmacol Rev* **64**: 676–705.

Chapter 2

Preanalytics and Quality Control of Different Substrates for Circulating DNA Studies

Fay Betsou and Wim Ammerlaan

Abstract

In this chapter, we review the most critical preanalytical factors in cirDNA analysis by sequencing, dPCR or BEAMing digital PCR, and methylation-specific PCR, with a focus on applications other than prenatal testing. We also review mitigation of preanalytical risks by the use of quality control procedures.

Introduction

cirDNA is used as a diagnostic, prognostic, or predictive biomarker. Diagnostic noninvasive prenatal testing (NIPT) routinely uses maternal and fetal cirDNA to test fetal aneuploidies via several available FDA-approved and CE-marked kits.[1,2] Analysis of cirDNA for clinical applications such as prognosis of cancer recurrence or metastasis, prediction of cancer therapy success, and adaptation of targeted therapies holds great promise.[3] cirDNA is being evaluated in cancer clinical trials as a biomarker and has already reached the stage of being used in clinical practice (e.g., by Guardant Health in the U.S. or Biocartis assays; https://www.genomeweb.com/pcr/ biocartis-gets-ce-marking-two-colorectal-cancer-liquid-biopsy-tests#.WvgVaGcR1vA). In disease areas other than cancer, such as nonalcoholic fatty liver disease (NAFL) and nonalcoholic steatohepatitis (NASH), the use of cirDNA as a diagnostic or prognostic biomarker is at the exploratory research stage, for example, in the clinical evolution of NAFL disease.[4] cirDNA methylation is also being explored as a biomarker in colorectal cancer[5] and NIPT,[6] and a diagnostic test for colorectal cancer based on the methylation of SEPTIN9[7,8] is already approved by FDA.

As for any biomarker, fitness for purpose of the specimens being used for cirDNA analysis is necessary for the accuracy of the analytical results.[9,10] Preanalytical handling and storage of blood, plasma, and purified cirDNA samples affect parameters such as DNA quantity, size distribution, and proportion of total DNA sample that is derived from the tumor. Uncontrolled and undocumented preanalytics may introduce catastrophic bias, invalidate clinical results, or lead to irreproducible research publications. Where samples collected from patients with a disease condition are compared to healthy control samples, it is particularly important that preanalytical variables such as blood storage and handling and also biobanking of plasma or cirDNA samples are standardized. This will often require advanced planning at the sample collection stage of a study.

Critical Preanalytical Factors

There are four major preanalytical factors that are critical for cirDNA extraction and preparation. The first critical factor is the processing of blood specimens, which carries two main challenges with regard to cirDNA extraction. The first challenge is the low concentration of around 1000 genome equivalents (GEs) per mL blood[11] cirDNA (a few ng per mL of plasma in healthy individuals), introducing the need for highest yield to ensure best sensitivity of downstream analysis. The second challenge with regard to cirDNA extraction is the possible "contamination" of cirDNA by bigger size cellular genomic DNA fragments, introducing the need for either prompt processing of blood samples, which is not always feasible in clinical settings, or for white blood cell (WBC) stabilization to ensure best specificity of downstream analysis.

With regard to blood collection, the question of serum versus plasma translates into the question of quantity or quality? Extraction of cirDNA consistently gives 5–8-fold higher yields in serum than in plasma.[12,13] Moreover, the team of Warton *et al.* have shown[13] that when blood collection tubes (BCT) are spiked with high-molecular-weight (MW) DNA, this spiked DNA is not recovered or detected electrophoretically in the serum cirDNA extracted from the blood collected in the tube. On the contrary, it is detected in its high-MW form in the plasma cirDNA extract, indicating that the spiked DNA may have been degraded during the serum processing. Therefore, the absence of high-MW DNA in cirDNA serum extracts may not guarantee the absence of contamination by cellular DNA fragments that may not be visible electrophoretically.

In another study evaluating cirDNA outputs in serum versus plasma, Parpart-Li *et al.* found significantly more total GEs, but significantly lower mutant allele fractions, in serum than in EDTA plasma from cancer patients. The fragment sizes in the cirDNA fraction extracted from serum ranged from 150 to 2000 bp, while the samples from plasma showed the single typical peak at around 150 bp.[14] Release of cellular DNA, therefore, seems to be taking place during the blood clotting process from lysing cells, thus explaining the higher yield of cirDNA obtained from serum. As a result, anticoagulated blood is the preferred option for any cirDNA-based assay. A summary of the studies having compared serum and plasma in the scope of cirDNA is shown in **Table 1**. A number of anticoagulant options for the collection of plasma exist, namely EDTA, citrate, and heparin. A 2014 survey of European laboratories showed that the overwhelming majority of studies that collect blood for cirDNA research use EDTA tubes, with only 2 out of 70 groups using sodium citrate tubes.[15] No group reported using heparin tubes, which may be due to concerns with residual heparin inhibiting downstream PCR applications.[16] EDTA has been shown to produce slower cell lysis than citrate or heparin,[17] and commercialized diagnostic kits require EDTA plasma as primary material.

Another important preanalytical factor for cirDNA collection is the time and temperature between blood collection and plasma isolation. Concerning the maximum allowable time between blood collection and processing by centrifugation for plasma separation, many biospecimen research studies indicate that EDTA blood should be processed in the 3–6 hr following collection, if it is stored at room temperature (RT). If EDTA blood is stored at 4°C, the delay can safely be extended to 8 hr[13] or to 24 hr.[14,18–23] **Table 2** summarizes cirDNA concentration kinetics in EDTA BCT.

In the event that prompt blood processing is not possible, the next question is whether the anticoagulated blood should be stabilized and with what type of stabilizer. The standard Paxgene tubes that have been used for years for blood cell nucleic-acid-based analyses are inadequate for cirDNA isolation because of extensive cell lysis.[24] Cell lysis also occurs in EDTA tubes, upon prolonged incubation of the blood, especially at RT. Following such WBC lysis, cellular genomic DNA fragments as well as DNases are

Table 1. Preanalytical Factors in Circulating DNA Extraction in Plasma and Serum

Ref	Plasma yield	Serum yield	Fold change	Plasma storage time	Serum clotting time	DNA extraction method	DNA quantification method
Lee et al. [50]	1×10^3 copies/mL	6×10^3 copies/mL	6x	2 hr	2 hr	HIV Monitor assay	Semi-qPCR (HLA-DQ)
Lui et al. [51]	1195.1 genome equivalent (GE)/mL	16344.8 GE/mL	14x	6-hr RT	6-hr RT	QIAamp Blood kit	qPCR (SKY, β-globin)
Thijssen et al. [52]	Healthy, 4.8 ± 3.6 ng/mL Cancer, 10.6 ± 14.2 ng/mL	Healthy, 12.9 ± 10.7 ng/mL Cancer, 47.4 ± 46.1 ng/mL	3x	<1 hr	<1 hr	Puregene (Gentra) +QIAquick PCR purification kit	qPCR (albumin) + Picogreen
Holdenrieder et al. [53]	~110 µg/L	~200 µg/L	2x	NA	NA	No extraction	CellDeath Detection ELISA
Warton et al. [13]	3.6 ± 0.5 ng/mL	32.7 ± 19.9 ng/mL	10x	30 min RT	30 min RT	QIAamp Circulating Nucleic Acids kit	qPCR (SFN1, SFTA3)
Ammerlaan et al. [12]	5 ± 0.5 ng/mL	23.6 ± 2.9 ng/mL	5x	5 min RT	45 min RT	QIAamp Circulating Nucleic Acids kit	Quant-IT Picogreen
Parpart-Li et al. [14]	~5000 GE/2 mL (size 155 bp)	~100,000 GE/2 mL (size 150–2000 bp)	20x	4-hr RT	30 min RT	QIAamp Circulating Nucleic Acids kit	Qubit HS assay + ddPCR (KRAS)

Table 2. Circulating DNA Concentration Kinetics (EDTA Blood Collection Tubes)

Ref	Baseline cirDNA	4 hr	8 hr	24 hr	48 hr	72 hr	120 hr	7 days	14 days
Lee et al.[50]	1×10^3 copies/mL	NA	NA	NA	NA	NA	NA	NA	3×10^4 copies/mL
Norton et al.[22]	~1000 copies/mL	NA	NA	stable	2x ↑	12x ↑	NA	49x ↑	204x ↑
Wong et al.[54]	Normalized medians (total genomic copies/mL)	NA	NA	1454	2631	NA	NA	7590	7995
Warton et al.[13]	4.4–4.9 ng/mL	stable	stable	6.5 ±2.2 ng/mL	10.8 ± 4.5 ng/mL	NA	NA	NA	NA
Parpart-Li et al.[14]	NA	NA	NA	~25x ↑ genome equivalent (GE)/mL	NA	NA	~500x ↑ GE/mL	~1300x ↑ GE/mL	NA
Warton et al.[55]	1.82–4.8 ng/mL	NA	NA	NA	NA	NA	NA	NA	57–98 ng/mL

released. While it has been shown that EDTA can inhibit endogenous DNase activity to some degree, DNA degradation may still occur.[25] Blood cell lysis is avoided by stabilization solutions, used in Streck, CellSave, Roche, Norgen Biotek, or Paxgene cirDNA tubes.[26–28] Stability claims of these products have generally been confirmed: 7 days at RT for Streck BCT and Paxgene cirDNA tubes. The stability of the cirDNA collection tube from Roche Diagnostics GmBH seems to be lower.[29] Yields and performance of cirDNA are comparable from Streck BCT and Paxgene cirDNA tubes (Ammerlaan, unpublished). Recently, an abstract from Qiagen showed that Streck tubes contain formaldehyde, which can induce DNA deaminations and introduce bias in cirDNA methylation analyses.[30] Furthermore, Paxgene cirDNA tubes allow unbiased quantification of methylated sequences to be performed and are therefore fit-for-purpose for downstream cirDNA methylation analyses.[31] **Table 3** summarizes comparison data between EDTA and the most commonly used BCT with stabilizers.

The consensus on plasma separation is for double spun plasma, with the second high-speed centrifugation at 16,000g before cirDNA extraction. However, while it is intuitive that a plasma centrifugation step will remove any WBC that were inadvertently collected and this can be visually corroborated with the observation of a pellet following the second spin, there is no published research that systematically examines the effects of plasma centrifugation to determine the optimum time and speed. A study examining the distribution of extracellular DNA in plasma vesicles reported an apoptotic body-associated DNA fraction that can be collected by a 1200g spin for 30 min.[32] It is of concern that this, and other microvesicle-associated fractions, may be removed during plasma centrifugation steps. A further consideration in plasma centrifugation is that non-DNA plasma components such

Table 3. Circulating DNA Preanalytical Factors in Most Commonly Used Blood Collection Tubes with Stabilizers

Ref	Endpoints (method)	Conditions	EDTA	Streck BCT	PAXgene cirDNA
Norton et al.[22]	Yield/size (ddPCR)	Up to 14 days RT	pDNA, 49x ↑ Day 7 and 204x ↑ Day 14 gDNA, 80x ↑ Day 7 and 456x ↑ Day 14	pDNA, stable Day 7 and 4x ↑ Day 14 gDNA, stable Day 7 and 2x ↑ Day 14	NA
Wong et al.[54]	Total and fetal copies/mL (FQA assay)	Up to 7 days at different temperatures	Fetal fraction ↓ Day 7, from 0.16 to 0.03	Fetal fraction stable Day 7, but ↓ at T°>32°C	NA
Parpart-Li et al.[14]	Genome equivalent (GE)/ mL (ddPCR) MAF (ddPCR)	Up to 7 days RT	1300% ↑ GE/mL 50%–100% ↓ GE/mL	6% ↑ GE/mL Stable	NA
Parpart-Li et al.[14]	GE/mL (ddPCR) MAF (ddPCR)	Up to 3 days 4°C	Stable 21% ↓ GE/mL	Stable 4% ↓ GE/mL	NA
Medina Diaz et al.[56]	Yield of short/long DNA fragments (qPCR) Mutational changes (BEAMing, SafeSeqS)	Up to 5 days RT, also 4°C and 40°C	NA	All endpoints stable, but ↑ long/short fragments from 0.2–0.3 to 0.5–0.6 at the extreme temperatures	NA
Warton et al.[55]	Yield (qPCR) size (qPCR+gel)	4 days RT	9–22x > yield 247 bp/115 bp ↑ High MW, intensively visible on gel	Stable yield 247 bp/115 bp ↓ High MW, just visible on gel	Stable yield 247 bp/115 bp ↑ No high MW on gel

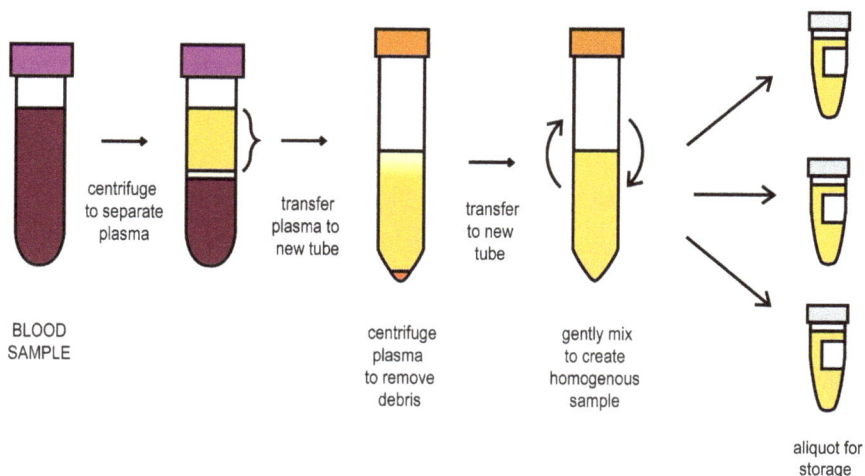

Fig. 1: Blood processing to create plasma aliquots for biobanking: double centrifugation removes contaminating cell debris; mixing the double-spun plasma prior to aliquoting creates uniform samples for reproducible results.

as lipids will form layers during the additional high-speed spin, and these layers will lead to nonuniform samples when the plasma is aliquoted directly from the centrifuged tube. The effect of this variation on cirDNA stability and extractability is not known. For this reason, some laboratories transfer the plasma to a fresh tube after the second spin, and mix it again, in order to obtain an even distribution of plasma components and uniform aliquots for long-term storage (**Fig. 1**) (Warton, pers. comm.).

The cirDNA extraction kit used is another critical preanalytical factor. Specific extraction methods are considered in detail in Chapter 4. In broad terms, standard genomic DNA extraction kits are unsuitable for cirDNA purification, as they are configured to bind high-MW DNA and exclude small-size fragments. This results in a purified sample that underrepresents the low-MW DNA that forms the bulk of cirDNA, resulting in an underestimate of the total cirDNA concentration, and an incorrect size distribution.

For downstream cirDNA methylation analyses, fitness-for-purpose of the cirDNA has been shown, although downstream analysis protocols may require modification.[13] If bisulfite conversion is used, the bisulfite conversion kit is another critical preanalytical factor. This methodology is covered in detail in Chapter 9.

The final critical preanalytical factor is cirDNA storage after extraction. Limited data have been published regarding the stability of cirDNA in storage. Sozzi and colleagues evaluated the stability of cirDNA in plasma stored at −80°C and of purified cirDNA stored at −20°C.[33] They found that storage of either sample type leads to a loss of cirDNA at a rate of about 30% per year. However, these data need to be considered in the light of subsequent advances in the understanding of cirDNA properties. Firstly, as no specialized cirDNA purification kit was commercially available at the time of that study, the authors used the QIAamp DNA Mini kit, which biases the purified sample against the low-MW fragments that form the bulk of the cirDNA pool. Hence, the 30% annual loss of cirDNA from frozen plasma may reflect the degradation of long DNA fragments more accurately than the degradation of short DNA fragments. Secondly, the purified DNA was eluted in water rather than buffer, and it is possible that acid hydrolysis of the unbuffered sample contributed to the 30% annual loss of DNA stored after extraction. Finally, stability data may not be transferrable between samples purified using different kits, as the final DNA sample likely contains different components (e.g., different elution buffer, carrier RNA vs. no carrier RNA, variation in contaminant carryover). No information regarding the influence of freeze-thaw cycles on sample stability is currently published.

Commercial protocols for whole genome amplification (WGA) from plasma are available (Sigma modified WGA2 or modified WGA4 protocols, https://www.sigmaaldrich.com/technical-documents/protocols/biology/whole-genome-amplification-serum-or-plasma.html); however, no independent validation has been published. cirDNA fragments of around 150 bp are too short for WGA by currently available methods (Johanna Trouet, unpublished).

A first set of evidence-based guidelines for processing specimens for cirDNA analyses has been published by El Messaoudi *et al.*[34] More evidence-based procedures and recommendations have been prepared by the European consortium CANCER-ID (https://www.cancer-id.eu/), in the context of the Innovative Medicines Initiative (IMI).[35] The European program SPIDIA (http://www.spidia.eu/) has developed a CEN Technical Specification standard for the preanalytical phase of cirDNA.[36] This standard includes requirements on the traceability of the most critical preanalytical factors.

Quality Control

Quality assurance of cirDNA processing methods includes method validation, documentation, internal quality control, and external quality control. A new ISO technical standard has been prepared by the ISO Technical Committee on Biotechnology (TC276), which includes requirements for validation of biospecimen processing methods.[37] This validation plan includes experimental plans for optimization of protocols relative to yield and purity of the produced cirDNA. It verifies fitness for purpose, feasibility, and the accuracy of specific downstream analyses, such as cirDNA sequencing. It sets the targets to be met for reproducibility and robustness to specific preanalytical variables, such as freeze-thaw cycles. Reproducibility and robustness are evaluated, based on selected analytical endpoints of scientific interest. These are usually quantitative, such as yield of cirDNA, size of cirDNA, or variant allele frequencies.

Recording and checking the preanalytical data associated with each sample via the Standard PREanalytical Code (SPREC) supports quality assurance and control. The latest version of the SPREC has been updated to include cirDNA-relevant options and codes.[38] More specifically, **Table 4** includes some of the options and corresponding codes that are relevant in cirDNA-related processing of samples.

Internal quality control of a processing method, such as cirDNA extraction, is performed through assays for biomarkers of

Table 4. Circulating DNA Processing and Corresponding Codes

Type of sample	
Blood (whole)	**BLD**
Plasma, single spin	**PL1**
Plasma, double spin	**PL2**
Serum	**SER**
Type of primary container	
Acid citrate dextrose	**ACD**
Chemical additives/stabilizers	ADD
Serum tube without clot activator	CAT
Citrate phosphate dextrose	**CPD**
EDTA and gel	EDG
Lithium heparin	**HEP**
Lithium heparin and gel	**LHG**
PAXgene® blood RNA+	**PAX**
Potassium EDTA	**PED**
PAXgene® blood DNA	PXD

Table 4.   (*Continued*)

Type of primary container		
RNA Later®		RNL
Sodium citrate		**SCI**
Non-aldehyde-based stabilizer for cell-free nucleic acids		SCK
Sodium EDTA		**SED**
Sodium heparin		SHP
Serum separator tube with clot activator		**SST**

Pre-centrifugation (delay between collection and processing)		
RT	<30 min	A1
2°C–10°C	<30 min	B1
RT	<2 hr	A
2°C–10°C	<2 hr	B
RT	2–4 hr	C
2°C–10°C	2–4 hr	D
RT	4–8 hr	E
2°C–10°C	4–8 hr	F
RT	8–12 hr	G
2°C–10°C	8–12 hr	H
RT	12–24 hr	I
2°C 10°C	12–24 hr	J
RT	24–48 hr	K
2°C–10°C	24–48 hr	L
RT	>48 hr	M
2°C–10°C	>48 hr	N

Centrifugation		
RT 10–15 min	<3000g no braking	A
RT 10– 15 min	<3000g with braking	B
2°C–10°C 10–15 min	<3000g no braking	C
2%–10°C 10–15 min	<3000g with braking	D

(*Continued*)

Table 4.   (*Continued*)

Second centrifugation		
RT 10–15 min	>10,000g with braking	I
2°C–10°C 10– 15 min	>10,000g with braking	J
Post-centrifugation delay		
<1 hr 2°C– 10°C		A
<1 hr RT		B
1–2 hr 2°C–10°C		C
1–2 hr RT		D
Long-term storage		
PP tube 0.5–2 mL	–85°C to –60°C	A
PP tube 0.5–2 mL	–35°C to (–18)°C	B
PP tube 0.5–2 mL	<–135°C	V
Cryotube 1–2 mL	LN	C
Cryotube 1–2 mL	–85°C to –60°C	D
Cryotube 1–2 mL	Programmable freezing to <–135°C	E
Plastic cryo straw	LN	F
Straw	–85°C to –60°C	G
Straw	–35°C to –18°C	H
Straw	Programmable freezing to <–135°C	I
PP tube ≥ 5 mL	–85°C to –60°C	J
PP tube ≥ 5 mL	–35°C to –18°C	K
Cryotube 1–2 mL	LN after temporary –85°C to –60°C	N

sample quality, such as electrophoretic assessment of cirDNA contamination by WBC DNA. Internal quality control is also achieved through usage of in-process quality control materials, such as spiked samples, which are processed in every extraction run. External quality control of a processing method is done through participation in corresponding external quality assurance processing schemes.

Analytical methods have their own set of internal quality control samples, which are tested in every run, such as a well-characterized cirDNA sample, and their own relevant external quality assurance testing schemes, such as quantification of cirDNA, or cirDNA sequencing and genotyping.

Internal Quality Controls

In-process QC Materials

Several spike-in sources can be applied. Synthetic ultramers, DNA fragments up 200 bases in length, represent an economical approach to the in-house production of in-process QC materials. Ultramers can be synthesized and contain any sequence/variant of interest and can be spiked in a blood tube that will undergo extraction in the same run with the plasma samples. However, synthetic ultramers are single-stranded naked DNA, and they do not anneal 100%; therefore, they do not wholly represent cirDNA. Alternatively, synthetic "gBlock Gene Fragments" can be designed. The "gBlock Gene Fragments" are synthetic dsDNA fragments ranging from 125 to 3000 bp. Synthesis allows for custom design sequences, for example, to create EGFR T790M and wt gBlocks in the cirDNA fragment size of approximately 150 bp, to be used as In-Process Controls (IPC). They have the advantage over the ultramers of being dsDNA, therefore not requiring annealing. More physiological and thus reflective of cirDNA is the ultrasonic shearing (e.g., Covaris) of purified DNA from appropriate cancer cell lines. This creates fragments of appropriate length (approximately 170 bp) and more natural sequence distribution by using the complete genome.

A disadvantage of these methods for in-process QC is that they produce naked DNA strands, which do not mimic the secondary structure of native cirDNA molecules, which are mononucleosomal DNA, in which the DNA is associated with histones. Mononucleosomal DNA preparations are, therefore, preferred as in-process QC materials. In the Integrated Biobank of Luxembourg (IBBL), such mononucleosomal DNA for spiking purposes is prepared from cell lines, with the following materials and method:

- A specific cancer cell line, as appropriate
- RPMI-1640 supplemented with 10% Fetal Bovine Serum (Gibco)
- PBS (Gibco)
- Trypsin (Lonza)
- Glycerol (Sigma)
- Nucleosome Preparation kit (Active Motif; cat# 53504)
- QIAquick PCR Purification Kits (QIAgen, cat# 28104)

Cells are collected with Trypsin and counted using CASY counter. Nucleosomes are prepared following the instruction manual from Active Motif (Nucleosome Preparation Kit; Version 1a, Active Motif). DNA is isolated from a part of the prepared nucleosomes, following the manufacturer's instruction (Nucleosome Preparation Kit; Version 1a, Active Motif). The Active Motif method for Mononucleosomes (MNs) preparations first isolates nuclei of a selected cell line or tissue, in the presence of protease inhibitors. The purified nuclei are digested by an Active Motif undisclosed enzymatic mixture, again in the presence of protease inhibitors. Digestion is stopped by adding EDTA. Prior to DNA quantification, the Mononucleosomal preparation is digested by Proteinase K, followed by a DNA cleanup with the QIAquick PCR purification kit. MN quantity equivalent to µg of DNA can be prepared from a single run starting with 10 million cells. The DNA is analyzed on a DNA high sensitivity HSD 5000 chip (4200 Tapestation) to verify the size is around 200 nucleotides and finally analyzed by dPCR for the mutations of interest.

Quality Control Assays

A review of relevant quality control assays for different types of biospecimens has been published by the ISBER Biospecimen Science Working group[39] and an online tool has been made available (www.findmyassay.com). Assays relevant to the context of cirDNA research are described as follows.

Quality of EDTA Plasma

The hemolytic index quantifies the level of hemoglobin in plasma. High levels of hemoglobin indicate hemolysis, that is, the lysis of red blood cells (RBCs). Although RBCs do not contain DNA and therefore there is no risk of contamination of the cirDNA fraction by RBC cellular DNA, hemolysis may indicate concomitant WBC lysis. The degree of hemolysis is measured either by hemoglobin ELISA, with a cutoff for significant hemolysis in plasma being 20 mg/L, or by simple spectrophotometric measurement at 414 nm with a cutoff for significant hemolysis being $OD_{414}>0.2$.[40]

When preanalytical data have not been documented, for example in the case of plasma legacy collections, the following quality control assays can be applied:

(i) Measurement of the Lacascore (ratio of ascorbic to lactic acid) in EDTA plasma can give an indication of the preanalytical quality of the plasma and more specifically indicates if the precentrifugation delay had been longer than 3 hr at RT.[41]

(ii) Measurement of IL-16 indicates if the precentrifugation delay of EDTA had been longer than 24 hr at RT (cutoff 313 pg/mL) or longer than 48 hr at RT (cutoff 897 pg/mL).[42]

Quality of Extracted cirDNA

Measurement of the concentration of extracted cirDNA can be done by high-sensitivity spectrofluorimetry or by qPCR or dPCR. A qPCR method targeting 90 bp and 222 bp fragments of LIPA2 has successfully been used for THE quantification of cirDNA in 1:40 diluted EDTA plasma, without previous extraction.[43] High-sensitivity microfluidic electrophoresis chips are used to assess contamination by high-MW cellular DNA.

A differential amplicon length PCR, such as the Kapa hgDNA quantification and QC kit, has been suggested as a relevant QC assay to assess the degree of contamination by high-MW cellular DNA. This kit amplifies the fragments of 41 bp, 129 bp, and 305 bp length, and a ratio of 305 bp/41 bp > 0.3 would be indicative of cell lysis.[29] Another differential amplicon PCR that can be used is an Alu qPCR with primer sets targeting fragments of 115 bp (Alu115) and 247 bp (Alu247). The cirDNA integrity can then be calculated as the ratio of Alu257/Alu115, which should be lower than 0.5.[44] A third differential amplicon dPCR assay that has been described is based on multiplex amplification of five single copy genomic loci of average length 71 bp and of four single copy loci of average length 471 bp. The cirDNA concentration was estimated as the difference between short amplicon-based GEs and long amplicon-based GEs.[45]

A qPCR targeting a genomic locus, present at one copy per haploid genome, such as *RPPH1*, *GAPDH*, *NAGK* or *ERV3*, can be used to measure extracted cirDNA copies/mL. However, more than one reference target should be used because the proportion of each locus in the cirDNA fraction is not necessarily the same as the corresponding proportion in cellular genomic DNA, with telomeric loci being more abundant in cirDNA.[46]

External Quality Controls

Proficiency Testing

IBBL has developed a proficiency testing program, which allows participating laboratories to assess the efficiency of their cirDNA extraction methods. The processing items that are distributed to participants are mononucleosomal DNA-spiked blood samples in Streck BCT or Paxgene cirDNA tubes.[47] Evaluation is based on cirDNA recovery and the presence or absence of contamination by high-MW genomic DNA.

The clinical laboratory EQA program providers AIOM, EMQN, ESP EQA, GenQA (part of UK NEQAS), and Gen&Tiss provide a pilot cirDNA EQA scheme to assess the standard of testing EGFR gene mutations in circulating free DNA in plasma (https://www.emqn.org/exciting-news-new-ctdna-scheme-plasma-testing-lung-cancer/).

Reference Materials

Reference materials are needed for formal analytical method validation according to ISO17025 accreditation requirements. There are only a few reference materials commercially available for these purposes.

Seracare commercialize a Seraseq™ circulating tumor DNA Reference Material. This is a mixture of human genomic DNA, fragmented into 170-bp fragments, in a commutable matrix (simulated plasma whose use is compatible with many different platforms and, therefore, allows comparison of different analytical platforms). The material contains several SNV and INDEL variants at allele frequencies of 5%–0.125%. The intended uses are targeted NGS, qPCR, and dPCR assays, and the Seraseq material can be used either as an internal QC material in the earlier mentioned assays or as an in-process QC material to monitor the performance of the extraction method as well as the performance of the analysis.

Horizon commercialize cirDNA HDx Reference Standards for method validation purposes (research use only). These materials are provided as mechanically sheared, fragmented DNA (average size 160 bp) from engineered human cell lines and contain variants at allelic frequencies down to 0.1%,[48] (https://www. horizondiscovery.com/media/resources/Application%20Notes/ reference-standards/independent-dPCR-study-of-horizon-cirDNA-reference-standards.pdf).

Devonshire *et al.* have developed and validated spike materials that allow users to measure cirDNA extraction efficiency, fragment size bias, and yield.[46] These materials are based on a linearized and digested plasmid, containing the *Arabidopsis thaliana* alcohol dehydrogenase gene (ADH) and fragments have sizes of 189 bp and roughly 3kb.

A homemade reference material that has been used for the analytical validation of a cirDNA NGS assay has been described and is based on overlapping extension PCR for site-directed mutagenesis to obtain fragments of 537–2030 bp, containing specific mutation sequences.[49]

Conclusion

The use of cirDNA as a biomarker has extended from NIPT to oncologic indications, and growing research and development efforts on cirDNA are targeting other disease areas. Standardization of the cirDNA preanalytical phase is key for the accuracy of analytical results and the reproducibility of research conclusions. The commercialization of BCT with stabilizers that avoid blood cell lysis has increased the robustness of cirDNA testing. External quality assurance programs for both cirDNA processing and analytical methods provide a means for laboratory benchmarking. Reference materials in combination with dPCR methods provide metrological traceability and the possibility of accreditation. With the mentioned developments, we are at a stage where we know which substrates to use, how to process them for each specific cirDNA-based application, and how to control for the quality of the substrates, of the cirDNA and of the methods applied.

References

1. Liu L, Li K, Fu X, *et al.* (2016) A forward look at noninvasive prenatal testing. *Trends Mol Med* **22**: 958–968.
2. Skrzypek H, Hui L. (2017) Noninvasive prenatal testing for fetal aneuploidy and single gene disorders. *Best Pract Res Clin Obstet Gynaecol* **42**: 26–38.
3. Cree IA, Uttley L, Buckley Woods H, *et al.* (2017) The evidence base for circulating tumour DNA blood-based biomarkers for the early detection of cancer: A systematic mapping review. *BMC Cancer* **17**: 697.
4. Karlas T, Weise L, Kuhn S, *et al.* (2017) Correlation of cell-free DNA plasma concentration with severity of non-alcoholic fatty liver disease. *J Transl Med* **15**: 106.
5. Worm Orntoft MB. (2018) Review of blood-based colorectal cancer screening: How far are circulating cell-free DNA methylation markers from clinical implementation? *Clin Colorectal Cancer* **17**: e415–e433.
6. Lim JH, Lee DE, Kim KS, *et al.* (2014) Non-invasive detection of fetal trisomy 21 using fetal epigenetic biomarkers with a high CpG density. *Clin Chem Lab Med* **52**: 641–647.
7. Potter NT, Hurban P, White MN, *et al.* (2014) Validation of a real-time PCR-based qualitative assay for the detection of methylated SEPT9 DNA in human plasma. *Clin Chem* **60**: 1183–1191.

8. Church TR, Wandell M, Lofton-Day C, *et al.* (2014) Prospective evaluation of methylated SEPT9 in plasma for detection of asymptomatic colorectal cancer. *Gut* **63**: 317–325.

9. Bartak BK, Kalmar A, Galamb O, *et al.* (2019) Blood collection and cell-free DNA isolation methods influence the sensitivity of liquid biopsy analysis for colorectal cancer detection. *Pathol Oncol Res* **25**: 915–923.

10. Bronkhorst AJ, Ungerer V, Diehl F, *et al.* (2020) Towards systematic nomenclature for cell-free DNA. *Hum Genet* **140**(4): 565–578.

11. Chiu RW, Poon LL, Lau TK, *et al.* (2001) Effects of blood-processing protocols on fetal and total DNA quantification in maternal plasma. *Clin Chem* **47**: 1607–1613.

12. Ammerlaan W, Trezzi JP, Lescuyer P, *et al.* (2014) Method validation for preparing serum and plasma samples from human blood for downstream proteomic, metabolomic, and circulating nucleic acid-based applications. *Biopreserv Biobank* **12**: 269–280.

13. Warton K, Lin V, Navin T, *et al.* (2014) Methylation-capture and next-generation sequencing of free circulating DNA from human plasma. *BMC Genomics* **15**: 476.

14. Parpart-Li S, Bartlett B, Popoli M, *et al.* (2017) The effect of preservative and temperature on the analysis of circulating tumor DNA. *Clin Cancer Res* **23**: 2471–2477.

15. Malentacchi F, Pizzamiglio S, Verderio P, *et al.* (2015) Influence of storage conditions and extraction methods on the quantity and quality of circulating cell-free DNA (ccfDNA): The SPIDIA-DNAplas external quality assessment experience. *Clin Chem Lab Med* **53**: 1935–1942.

16. Farnert A, Arez AP, Correia AT, *et al.* (1999) Sampling and storage of blood and the detection of malaria parasites by polymerase chain reaction. *Trans R Soc Trop Med Hyg* **93**: 50–53.

17. Lam NY, Rainer TH, Chiu RW, Lo YM. (2004) EDTA is a better anticoagulant than heparin or citrate for delayed blood processing for plasma DNA analysis. *Clin Chem* **50**: 256–257.

18. Xue X, Teare MD, Holen I, *et al.* (2009) Optimizing the yield and utility of circulating cell-free DNA from plasma and serum. *Clin Chim Acta* **404**: 100–104.

19. Page K, Guttery DS, Zahra N, *et al*. (2013) Influence of plasma processing on recovery and analysis of circulating nucleic acids. *PLoS One* **8**: e77963.

20. Jung M, Klotzek S, Lewandowski M, *et al*. (2003) Changes in concentration of DNA in serum and plasma during storage of blood samples. *Clin Chem* **49**: 1028–1029.

21. Board RE, Williams VS, Knight L, *et al*. (2008) Isolation and extraction of circulating tumor DNA from patients with small cell lung cancer. *Ann N Y Acad Sci* **1137**: 98–107.

22. Norton SE, Lechner JM, Williams T, Fernando MR. (2013) A stabilizing reagent prevents cell-free DNA contamination by cellular DNA in plasma during blood sample storage and shipping as determined by digital PCR. *Clin Biochem* **46**: 1561–1565.

23. Barrett AN, Zimmermann BG, Wang D, *et al*. (2011) Implementing prenatal diagnosis based on cell-free fetal DNA: Accurate identification of factors affecting fetal DNA yield. *PLoS One* **6**: e25202.

24. Toro PV, Erlanger B, Beaver JA, *et al*. (2015) Comparison of cell stabilizing blood collection tubes for circulating plasma tumor DNA. *Clin Biochem* **48**: 993–998.

25. Barra GB, Santa Rita TH, de Almeida Vasques J, *et al*. (2015) EDTA-mediated inhibition of DNases protects circulating cell-free DNA from ex vivo degradation in blood samples. *Clin Biochem* **48**: 976–981.

26. van Dessel LF, Beije N, Helmijr JC, *et al*. (2017) Application of circulating tumor DNA in prospective clinical oncology trials - standardization of preanalytical conditions. *Mol Oncol* **11**: 295–304.

27. Sherwood JL, Corcoran C, Brown H, *et al*. (2016) Optimised pre-analytical methods improve KRAS mutation detection in circulating tumour DNA (ctDNA) from patients with non-small cell lung cancer (NSCLC). *PLoS One* **11**: e0150197.

28. Kang Q, Henry NL, Paoletti C, *et al*. (2016) Comparative analysis of circulating tumor DNA stability In K3EDTA, Streck, and CellSave blood collection tubes. *Clin Biochem* **49**: 1354–1360.

29. Nikolaev S, Lemmens L, Koessler T, *et al*. (2018) Circulating tumoral DNA: Preanalytical validation and quality control in a diagnostic laboratory. *Anal Biochem* **542**: 34–39.

30. Groelz D, Viertler C, Pabst D, *et al.* (2018) Impact of storage conditions on the quality of nucleic acids in paraffin embedded tissues. *PLoS One* **13**: e0203608.

31. Schmidt B, Reinicke D, Reindl I, *et al.* (2017) Liquid biopsy—Performance of the PAXgene(R) blood ccfDNA tubes for the isolation and characterization of cell-free plasma DNA from tumor patients. *Clin Chim Acta* **469**: 94–98.

32. Lazaro-Ibanez E, Sanz-Garcia A, Visakorpi T, *et al.* (2014) Different gDNA content in the subpopulations of prostate cancer extracellular vesicles: Apoptotic bodies, microvesicles, and exosomes. *Prostate* **74**: 1379–1390.

33. Sozzi G, Roz L, Conte D, *et al.* (2005) Effects of prolonged storage of whole plasma or isolated plasma DNA on the results of circulating DNA quantification assays. *J Natl Cancer Inst* **97**: 1848–1850.

34. El Messaoudi S, Rolet F, Mouliere F, Thierry AR. (2013) Circulating cell free DNA: Preanalytical considerations. *Clin Chim Acta* **424**: 222–230.

35. Lampignano R, Neumann MHD, Weber S, *et al.* (2020) Multicenter evaluation of circulating cell-free DNA extraction and downstream analyses for the development of standardized (Pre)analytical work flows. *Clin Chem* **66**: 149–160.

36. CEN/TS 16835-3 Venous Whole Blood - Part 3: Isolated circulating cell free DNA from plasma 2015.

37. ISO 21899:2020 Biotechnology – Biobanking – General requirements for the validation and verification of processing methods for biological material in biobanks.

38. Betsou F, Bilbao R, Case J, *et al.* (2018) Standard PREanalytical code version 3.0. *Biopreserv Biobank* **16**: 9–12.

39. Betsou F, Bulla A, Cho SY, *et al.* (2016) Assays for qualification and quality stratification of clinical Biospecimens used in research: A technical report from the ISBER Biospecimen science working group. *Biopreserv Biobank* **14**: 398–409.

40. Appierto V, Callari M, Cavadini E, *et al.* (2014) A lipemia-independent NanoDrop((R))-based score to identify hemolysis in plasma and serum samples. *Bioanalysis* **6**: 1215–1226.

41. Trezzi JP, Bulla A, Bellora C, *et al.* (2016) LacaScore: A novel plasma sample quality control tool based on ascorbic acid and lactic acid levels. *Metabolomics* **12**: 96.

42. Kofanova O, Henry E, Aguilar Quesada R, *et al.* (2018) IL8 and IL16 levels indicate serum and plasma quality. *Clin Chem Lab Med* **56**: 1054–1062.

43. Breitbach S, Tug S, Helmig S, *et al.* (2014) Direct quantification of cell-free, circulating DNA from unpurified plasma. *PLoS One* **9**: e87838.

44. Fawzy A, Sweify KM, El-Fayoumy HM, Nofal N. (2016) Quantitative analysis of plasma cell-free DNA and its DNA integrity in patients with metastatic prostate cancer using ALU sequence. *J Egypt Natl Canc Inst* **28**: 235–242.

45. Markus H, Contente-Cuomo T, Farooq M, *et al.* (2018) Evaluation of pre-analytical factors affecting plasma DNA analysis. *Sci Rep* **8**: 7375.

46. Devonshire AS, Whale AS, Gutteridge A, *et al.* (2014) Towards standardisation of cell-free DNA measurement in plasma: Controls for extraction efficiency, fragment size bias and quantification. *Anal Bioanal Chem* **406**: 6499–6512.

47. Gaignaux A, Ashton G, Coppola D, *et al.* (2016) A biospecimen proficiency testing program for biobank accreditation: Four years of experience. *Biopreserv Biobank* **14**: 429–439.

48. Amit H, Wei SH, Armisen-Garrido J, *et al.* (2015) Using cell free DNA reference standards to evaluate the analytical performance of circulating tumor DNA testing and solid organ transplant health surveillance. *BioTechniques* **59**: 248–250.

49. Yang X, Chu Y, Zhang R, *et al.* (2017) Technical validation of a next-generation sequencing assay for detecting clinically relevant levels of breast cancer-related single-nucleotide variants and copy number variants using simulated cell-free DNA. *J Mol Diagn* **19**: 525–536.

50. Lee TH, Montalvo L, Chrebtow V, Busch MP. (2001) Quantitation of genomic DNA in plasma and serum samples: Higher concentrations of genomic DNA found in serum than in plasma. *Transfusion* **41**: 276–282.

51. Lui YY, Chik KW, Chiu RW, *et al.* (2002) Predominant hematopoietic origin of cell-free DNA in plasma and serum after sex-mismatched bone marrow transplantation. *Clin Chem* **48**: 421–427.

52. Thijssen MA, Swinkels DW, Ruers TJ, de Kok JB. (2002) Difference between free circulating plasma and serum DNA in patients with colorectal liver metastases. *Anticancer Res* **22**: 421–425.

53. Holdenrieder S, Stieber P, Chan LY, *et al.* (2005) Cell-free DNA in serum and plasma: comparison of ELISA and quantitative PCR. *Clin Chem* **51**: 1544–1546.

54. Wong D, Moturi S, Angkachatchai V, *et al.* (2013) Optimizing blood collection, transport and storage conditions for cell free DNA increases access to prenatal testing. *Clin Biochem* **46**: 1099–1104.

55. Warton K, Yuwono NL, Cowley MJ, *et al.* (2017) Evaluation of streck BCT and PAXgene stabilised blood collection tubes for cell-free circulating DNA studies in plasma. *Mol Diagn Ther* **21**: 563–570.

56. Medina Diaz I, Nocon A, Mehnert DH, *et al.* Performance of streck cfDNA blood collection tubes for liquid biopsy testing. *PLoS One* **11**: e0166354.

Chapter 3

Considerations in Biobanking Blood Samples and Plasma Volume for Circulating DNA Studies

Kate Mahon, Goli Samimi and Kristina Warton

Abstract

Clinical circulating DNA studies are contingent on the availability of appropriate biospecimens and linked patient data. Incorporating circulating DNA analysis in clinical trial design adds value to the trial, as well as allowing future retrospective analysis of markers that may be unknown at the time of the trial. However, this requires forward planning and commitment to sample curation. This chapter considers circulating DNA in the broader context of biobanking.

How much plasma does this assay need? If not the first question in a circulating DNA study, it is perhaps the one asked with the most consternation. Unless project-specific, prospective biobanking is undertaken, the volumes of clinical plasma samples available for circulating DNA studies are often small. This chapter also examines the implications of the typically low biological circulating DNA concentrations and provides an overview of the plasma volumes used in circulating DNA research in cancer.

Considerations in Biobanking Blood Samples for Studies of Circulating DNA in Plasma

Biobanking involves collection, storage, maintenance, and analysis of biological samples and clinical data for future clinical and research purposes.[1] In recent years, biobanking has become a standard requirement for clinical trials and is increasingly identified as an ideal standard for routine clinical care. While this is an admirable goal, multiple issues arise in such large-scale collections and biobank procedures must be well researched and planned from the outset.

As the number and scale of biobanks has expanded over recent years, it has become imperative to define and classify biobanks. Many classification systems have been developed, and with the complexity and evolution of biobanking, these classification systems are likely to evolve with time. A detailed classification system including multiple elements proposed by Watson and Barnes[2] has been adopted internationally. This schema utilizes four functional elements to define individual biobanks. These are:

1. Donor/participant — describes the defining features of the test subjects such as disease state (healthy/at risk/specific disease), alive or deceased, age categorization.
2. Design — including accrual plan (prospective/retrospective), collection timepoints (single/multiple), scale (single or multiple research studies), extent of linked data collection.
3. Biospecimens — including type of biospecimen (e.g., blood, tissue, fluid, cells), method of preservation.

4. Brand — including leadership (researchers, groups, institutions), sponsors and users (single, several, or many).

The elements broadly detailed in this classification schema highlight the need to consider and define these aspects in the optimal design and setup of a biobank to ensure that it is optimally fit for purpose from the outset.

Purpose of Biobank

The specific purpose of a biobank should be the initial consideration. Biobanks for circulating tumor DNA (ctDNA) may focus on early detection and diagnosis of cancer, detecting disease recurrence in patients following curative intent treatment, or predicting and/or monitoring response to therapy. This purpose will define the study population, location, and method of accrual. The timing of sample collection is also an important consideration. Clearly, this must fit the proposed purpose of the test but must also be practical in the clinical setting. Inconvenient sampling such as requiring patients to attend for tests when they would not normally do so or at multiple time points will hamper the ability to recruit and retain study subjects. Furthermore, if a test proves to be clinically useful, translation into clinical practice will be challenging if the testing procedure is complicated and impractical.

Ideally, the scale of a biobank and the proposed number of users should also be defined from the outset. The number of users can range from a single research group or institution to multiple groups across international sites. With greater numbers of users and sites, the need for clearly detailed standardized operating procedures (SOPs) for specimen collection and processing and considered data management becomes particularly important. Large biobanks may require samples to be moved long distances for storage and these procedures also need to be thoroughly detailed to avoid degradation of samples. Recognition that preanalytical inconsistencies may cause greater variability in results than the true biological differences[3] has led to standardized frameworks (including Standard PREanalytical Code[4] and Biospecimen Reporting for Improved Study Quality[5]) to ensure thorough documentation and reporting of essential elements of preanalytical processing. A sample processing trail (e.g., dates, times, temperature, location, operator) should be detailed to flag any potential issues in sample quality.[6] Reliable labeling systems to track sample locations are imperative to avoid lost or misidentified samples. Ongoing investigator training and audit procedures are also required to maintain consistency. International organizations such as the National Cancer Institute (NCI) provide best practice documents encompassing small to very large scale biobanks to guide essential aspects of setup and management.[7] While ensuring best practice, complying with internationally recognized protocols may also facilitate collaboration and integration with other biobanks in the future.

Ethical Considerations

Ethical considerations and informed consent are paramount in biobank management, particularly in the proposed genetic analysis of stored samples. International biobanks include an extra layer of complexity with a wide range of legal requirements in different jurisdictions. Difficulties arise when the nature of a proposed test cannot clearly be defined at the time of consent. Obtaining consent for each new research project arising from a biobank is impractical and often impossible so a "broad consent" encompassing as yet unspecified future uses is required. The legal and ethical implications of such a consent have long been debated.[8] The range of consent procedures in biobanks internationally is wide.[9] Many biobank consent procedures allow subjects to specify exactly how their specimens may be used including genetic testing and future unspecified research. Consent processes should inform subjects about long-term storage of samples and potential sharing of data and specimens with other researchers. Confidentiality procedures must also be clearly detailed such as de-identification of samples and clinical data including how data may be shared with other research groups (e.g., aggregated data versus individual patient data). While most patient information includes details around the physical risks of sample collection (e.g., venipuncture or biopsy), potential legal and psychosocial risks associated with possible results should also be communicated. Patient access to genetic information arising from study results must be considered. Genomic findings may not only impact the subject but may also have implications for family members. Plans to communicate positive results back to participants or family members must be determined and should be clearly explained at the time of consent. Obligations around reporting results to external organizations (e.g., government agencies, insurance companies) must also be detailed.[10]

Clinical Data

Accurate, thorough, and accessible clinical data management is crucial for the analysis of accompanying biospecimens. A minimum clinical data set should be ascertained at the outset and data collection time points should be established. In some instances, clinical data will only need to be documented at the time of specimen collection; however, most cancer research will benefit from ongoing followup. Clear plans must be made around when, how, and by whom ongoing clinical details will be obtained (e.g., at specific clinic visits, by phone call or mail outs). Dedicated staff are usually required to obtain long-term follow-up data and maintain database integrity.

Reliable, flexible, and secure information technology systems are imperative. Clinical data should be linked with biospecimen collection information and results of analyses. Ideally, databases will be easily accessible by all relevant members of the research team and will allow extraction of data, which may be usefully shared between research groups for future collaboration. Maintaining data accessibility, such as in web-based systems, while ensuring data security to maintain patient confidentiality, is an additional challenge. Defined security levels are required so that users can only access the information required for their specific tasks and research sites. While multiple systems are available, both commercially and through academic institutions, no system provides a perfect comprehensive solution. Future integration of biobank databases may be better facilitated by standardization of minimum data sets, ontologies, and data formats.[10]

Considerations in Selecting Assay Plasma Volume

When considering biobanking of plasma for circulating DNA (cirDNA) studies, collecting an adequate volume can maximize the usefulness of the samples for downstream analysis. The volume of plasma needed for a biomarker assay is a key question when designing experiments or planning clinical studies. Too little, and there won't be enough DNA target for reliable detection; too much, and the reaction may be crippled by blood-derived enzyme inhibitors. This issue is particularly pertinent when designing assays intended for the early diagnosis of cancer, where detection of very low concentrations of target, corresponding to very low tumor volume, is required for the assay to be clinically useful.

The optimal volume of plasma for an assay or a protocol is dependent on a number of factors; these being the total volume of plasma available, the concentration of tumor-derived DNA in the plasma, the sensitivity of the detection assay, and the presence of blood-derived inhibitors. We will consider each of these in turn, with a focus on PCR, since it is the most commonly used detection method, and underpins many other types of molecular analyses (e.g., sequencing).

Available Plasma Volume

Limitations stemming from the volume of available plasma are the easiest to consider. Blood samples collected from patients in a clinical context are generally quite low volume, with a single large-draw blood tube yielding at best around 10 mL of blood and 5 mL of plasma, while standard blood tubes yield around 4 mL of blood and 2 mL of plasma. Unless the blood collection is specifically carried out for a particular project, the sample may be further split between different studies. The challenge is more acute for rare cancer types, since a small number of biospecimens means that less sample is spread between projects. Another issue arises when blood from patients is being compared against healthy controls for the purpose of biomarker discovery or validation, as an equivalent volume of matched control sample needs to be available. In addition to the work of collecting, processing, and storing the plasma, patient samples also require the collection and curation of sample-linked clinical information. All in all, this makes patient plasma samples a much valued and limited resource.

The low volume of plasma available can be a hurdle to biomarker development. Volumes of 500 µL or less are reported in studies, presumably reflecting the amount of biobanked sample that could be obtained.[11–13] Early stages of biomarker development are most likely to be carried out on retrospective biobanked samples,[14] since early stage biomarker discovery is considered risky and generally not seen to warrant a prospective plasma collection effort. Ironically, it is the early stages that often require the most plasma, in particular if they involve repeated measurements or evaluation of multiple biomarker candidates to identify ones that have adequate sensitivity and specificity.[15] Publicly funded biobanks may be unwilling to release large volumes of plasma for early stage testing of unvalidated biomarkers. Thus, a situation arises where the largest number of biomarker candidates needs to be tested at the project stage where the lowest volume of plasma is readily available.

The highest volume of plasma will be available from patients once the test is utilized in a clinical setting, and a similarly large volume will be available from samples collected in any prospective trials planned as part of biomarker validation, in which the entire blood sample can be allocated for the study. The question then is whether to design assays based on the volume of patient plasma that will be available from individual patients in a clinical setting or based on the likely more limited volume of plasma that will be available to validate the biomarker in retrospective cohorts. This question can only be answered within the practical and budget constraints of each individual project and depends largely on the funds allocated to sourcing or collecting biospecimens.

Concentration of cirDNA in Plasma

The concentration of cirDNA in plasma has been noted to vary widely, even in healthy individuals,[16] and determination of the true concentration is hampered by samples being particularly sensitive to handling and measurement artefacts. For example, storage of collected blood prior to plasma separation leads to lysis of leukocyte and contamination of the cirDNA pool with leukocyte genomic DNA, thus increasing the apparent concentration.[17,18] A large, multi-center study prospectively examining the relationship between cirDNA concentration and cancer risk identified the research center carrying out the blood collection and processing as by far the single most influential variable in determining cirDNA levels, demonstrating the impact that handling protocols have on derivation of cirDNA.[19] In addition to the effects of sample handling, different extraction methods have large differences in yield,[20–22] inevitably leading to differences in apparent cirDNA concentration reported by studies applying the different methodologies. There is also some indication that cirDNA in plasma and purified DNA samples degrade during storage, further decreasing the substrate available for analysis.[23,24] From the perspective of healthy variation, physical activity has profound effects on cfDNA levels, with transient increases of up to ninefold observed immediately after exercise.[25]

Quantitation of cirDNA from Plasma

There is a range of techniques available to quantitate cirDNA purified from plasma. These include spectrophotometry-based techniques such as Nanodrop (ThermoFisher), techniques that rely on fluorescent dye binding such as Picogreen Kit and the Picogreen-based QuBit fluorometer (both from ThermoFisher), and various types of qPCR. The different quantitation methods produce different concentration results. For example, QuBit has been shown to measure around several-fold the apparent yield of qPCR,[26] most likely due to PCR not detecting DNA fragments below the size of the target amplicon. For the purposes of this chapter, we will consider the quantity of cirDNA in plasma to refer to the quantity of DNA that is detectable by PCR, since this is the amount accessible to analysis by PCR-based methods. While this introduces some consistency, there is still a level of artefactual variation, since the fragmented nature of cirDNA means that using a shorter PCR assay results in a higher apparent cirDNA concentration[27] (see Chapter 5), and the positioning of nucleosomes relative to the PCR amplicon is also important.[28,29]

With the above considerations in mind, most current estimates place the cirDNA concentration in healthy individuals between 1 and 10 ng per milliliter of plasma.[30] The level in cancer patients is higher, with the increase due to tumor DNA as well as an increased contribution from nontumor cells.[31] The proportion of total cirDNA derived from the tumor depends on the tumor volume and stage,[31,32] and possibly on the type of cancer.[33] The upper end of the range, measured in advanced tumors, can be quite high, with the most tumor DNA-rich samples containing ~65% ctDNA in cirDNA from advanced ovarian cancer patients,[33] 27% in patients with metastatic colorectal cancer,[31] and ~90% in breast cancer.[34] Different subclones of tumor can contribute different amounts of ctDNA. For example, Murtaza and colleagues found that mutations already present in the primary tumor of a breast cancer patient ranged from 3.8% to 34.9% in plasma sampled at multiple time points over ~16 months, while mutations limited to metastatic tumor deposits ranged from 2.5% to 19% over the same time period.[35] Evidently, the lower range of ctDNA concentration in cancer patients cannot be determined below the sensitivity of the analysis techniques applied, but mutant allele fractions of 0.01% have been measured in early stage colorectal cancer patients by a variation on digital PCR technique (BEAM-ing — Beads Emulsion Amplification and Magnetics)[31] and by massively parallel sequencing.[36]

The cirDNA concentration, together with the ctDNA fraction, allows some estimate of the ctDNA amount available for an assay and thus of the minimum plasma input requirements for an assay of a given sensitivity. For example, with 10 ng of cirDNA per milliliter, and 5% tumor DNA, an assay needs to detect 500 pg of target when 1 mL of plasma is used, and with 0.5% tumor DNA it needs to detect 50 pg of target. Numbers of ctDNA molecules in plasma samples from cancer patients have been directly quantitated by sequencing, with techniques able to detect less than 1 mutant molecule per milliliter of plasma.[32,36] For some applications, detecting the smallest possible ctDNA amount is less important than for others. For example, ctDNA assays can be applied to patient monitoring during drug treatment, without stringent sensitivity requirements. This variable application is analogous to protein biomarkers, where sensitivity and specificity requirements for cancer monitoring are much less stringent than for cancer diagnosis. For example, CA125 and CEA are routinely used for ovarian and colorectal cancer patient monitoring respectively but are unsuitable for use in diagnostic cancer screening.[37–39]

Reporting Standards

Consistency in reporting cfDNA studies has repeatedly been called for in the field to allow interpretation and replication.[40] Where authors do not explicitly state the plasma volume corresponding to a particular amount of cirDNA used in a PCR or other downstream assay, and it is not always possible to calculate it from the methods information provided. In order to allow readers to calculate the volume of plasma effectively analyzed in each assay, the authors need to provide the following information: volume of plasma used in the cirDNA extraction; DNA elution/resuspension volume; and the seeding volume of the PCR. Where the DNA is bisulfite converted and used for methylation analysis, authors also need to provide the volume of purified DNA used in the bisulfite conversion reaction, and the elution/resuspension volume of the bisulfite-converted DNA, followed by the PCR seeding volume. Where the methods of published studies describe only the total amount (i.e., nano- or picograms) of cirDNA that was used in a PCR reaction, it may not be possible to calculate back to the corresponding volume of plasma without the plasma concentration of cirDNA also being provided. Unfortunately, in published research papers, the necessary information about plasma volumes used and recovered at each step during cirDNA extraction/conversion is the exception rather than the rule.

Blood-Derived PCR Inhibitors

If the volume of plasma used as starting material in an assay is not limited by the total amount of plasma available, then it may be limited by the carryover of blood-derived PCR inhibitors. PCR inhibitors are the compounds present in a sample that have either carried over from the biospecimen extracted or been introduced during DNA purification or bisulfite treatment. Blood-derived PCR inhibitors include hemoglobin and immunoglobulin G,[41,42] while introduced inhibitors include heparin, ethanol, and detergent.[43,44]

For this reason, provided there is a sufficient volume of plasma available, choosing a purification method that halves the carryover of PCR inhibitors is as good as doubling the yield from the purification protocol, as it would allow the PCR reaction to be seeded with double the amount of eluted DNA without encountering the problem of inhibitors.

Summary

Biobanks provide opportunities for identifying circulating DNA mutations for diagnosis, prognosis, and therapeutic decision-making. Circulating DNA mutations can be difficult to identify, often occurring in small numbers of individuals and across cancer types. Integration of biobanks can overcome this issue to increase patient numbers and allow analysis of data across tumor-specific collections. Biobanking adequate plasma volumes will help to maximize the usefulness of the samples. To avoid the multitude of issues that may arise, thorough planning and consideration of biobank procedures at the outset are essential.

References

1. Smith ME, Aufox S. (2013) Biobanking: The melding of research with clinical care. *Curr Genet Med Rep* **1**: 122–128.
2. Watson PH, Barnes RO. (2011) A proposed schema for classifying human research biobanks. *Biopreserv Biobank* **9**: 327–333.
3. Ellervik C, Vaught J. (2015) Preanalytical variables affecting the integrity of human biospecimens in biobanking. *Clin Chem* **61**: 914–934.
4. Betsou F, Lehmann S, Ashton G, *et al.* (2010) Standard preanalytical coding for biospecimens: Defining the sample PREanalytical code. *Cancer Epidemiol Biomarkers Prev* **19**: 1004–1011.
5. Moore HM, Kelly AB, Jewell SD, *et al.* (2011) Biospecimen reporting for improved study quality (BRISQ). *Cancer Cytopathol* **119**: 92–101.
6. Vaught J, Abayomi A, Peakman T, *et al.* (2014) Critical issues in international biobanking. *Clin Chem* **60**: 1368–1374.
7. Insititute NC. (2016) *NCI Best Practices for Biospecimen Resources*.

8. Hansson MG, Dillner J, Bartram CR, *et al.* (2006) Should donors be allowed to give broad consent to future biobank research? *Lancet Oncol* **7**: 266–269.

9. Wolf LE, Bouley TA, McCulloch CE. (2010) Genetic research with stored biological materials: Ethics and practice. *IRB* **32**: 7–18.

10. Watson RW, Kay EW, Smith D. (2010) Integrating biobanks: Addressing the practical and ethical issues to deliver a valuable tool for cancer research. *Nat Rev Cancer* **10**: 646–651.

11. Olsson E, Winter C, George A, *et al.* (2015) Serial monitoring of circulating tumor DNA in patients with primary breast cancer for detection of occult metastatic disease. *EMBO Mol Med* **7**: 1034–1047.

12. Alborelli I, Generali D, Jermann P, *et al.* (2019) Cell-free DNA analysis in healthy individuals by next-generation sequencing: A proof of concept and technical validation study. *Cell Death Dis* **10**: 534.

13. Zemmour H, Planer D, Magenheim J, *et al.* (2018) Non-invasive detection of human cardiomyocyte death using methylation patterns of circulating DNA. *Nat Commun* **9**: 1443.

14. Mahon KL, Qu W, Devaney J, *et al.* (2014) Methylated Glutathione S-transferase 1 (mGSTP1) is a potential plasma free DNA epigenetic marker of prognosis and response to chemotherapy in castrate-resistant prostate cancer. *Br J Cancer* **111**: 1802–1809.

15. Lofton-Day C, Model F, Devos T, *et al.* (2008) DNA methylation biomarkers for blood-based colorectal cancer screening. *Clin Chem* **54**: 414–423.

16. Thierry AR, El Messaoudi S, Gahan PB, *et al.* (2016) Origins, structures, and functions of circulating DNA in oncology. *Cancer Metastasis Rev* **35**: 347–376.

17. El Messaoudi S, Rolet F, Mouliere F, Thierry AR. (2013) Circulating cell free DNA: Preanalytical considerations. *Clin Chim Acta* **424**: 222–230. doi:10.1016/j.cca.2013.05.022. Epub May 30.

18. Warton K, Lin V, Navin T, *et al.* (2014) Methylation-capture and next-generation sequencing of free circulating DNA from human plasma. *BMC Genomics* **15**: 476. doi:10.1186/471-2164-15-476.

19. Gormally E, Hainaut P, Caboux E, *et al.* (2004) Amount of DNA in plasma and cancer risk: A prospective study. *Int J Cancer* **111**: 746–749.

20. Diefenbach RJ, Lee JH, Kefford RF, Rizos H. (2018) Evaluation of commercial kits for purification of circulating free DNA. *Cancer Genet* **228–229**: 21–7.

21. Devonshire AS, Whale AS, Gutteridge A, *et al*. (2014) Towards standardisation of cell-free DNA measurement in plasma: Controls for extraction efficiency, fragment size bias and quantification. *Anal Bioanal Chem* **406**: 6499–6512.

22. Warton K, Graham LJ, Yuwono N, Samimi G. (2018) Comparison of 4 commercial kits for the extraction of circulating DNA from plasma. *Cancer Genet* **228–229**: 143–150.

23. Sozzi G, Roz L, Conte D, *et al*. (2005) Effects of prolonged storage of whole plasma or isolated plasma DNA on the results of circulating DNA quantification assays. *J Natl Cancer Inst* **97**: 1848–1850.

24. Sato A, Nakashima C, Abe T, *et al*. Investigation of appropriate pre-analytical procedure for circulating free DNA from liquid biopsy. *Oncotarget* **9**: 31904–31914.

25. de Sousa MV, Madsen K, Fukui R, *et al*. Carbohydrate supplementation delays DNA damage in elite runners during intensive microcycle training. *Eur J Appl Physiol* **112**: 493–500.

26. Ponti G, Maccaferri M, Manfredini M, *et al*. (2018) The value of fluorimetry (Qubit) and spectrophotometry (NanoDrop) in the quantification of cell-free DNA (cfDNA) in malignant melanoma and prostate cancer patients. *Clin Chim Acta* **479**: 14–19.

27. Andersen RF, Spindler KL, Brandslund I, *et al*. (2015) Improved sensitivity of circulating tumor DNA measurement using short PCR amplicons. *Clin Chim Acta* **439**: 97–101.

28. Snyder MW, Kircher M, Hill AJ, *et al*. (2016) Cell-free DNA comprises an in vivo nucleosome footprint that informs its tissues-of-origin. *Cell* **164**: 57–68.

29. Johansson G, Andersson D, Filges S, *et al*. (2019) Considerations and quality controls when analyzing cell-free tumor DNA. *Biomol Detect Quantif* **17**: 100078.

30. Wan JCM, Massie C, Garcia-Corbacho J, *et al*. (2017) Liquid biopsies come of age: Towards implementation of circulating tumour DNA. *Nat Rev Cancer* **17**: 223–238.

31. Diehl F, Li M, Dressman D, *et al*. (2005) Detection and quantification of mutations in the plasma of patients with colorectal tumors. *Proc Natl Acad Sci USA* **102**: 16368–16373.

32. Bettegowda C, Sausen M, Leary RJ, *et al*. (2014) Detection of circulating tumor DNA in early- and late-stage human malignancies. *Sci Transl Med* **6**: 224ra224.

33. Forshew T, Murtaza M, Parkinson C, *et al*. (2012) Noninvasive identification and monitoring of cancer mutations by targeted deep sequencing of plasma DNA. *Sci Transl Med* **4**: 136ra168.

34. Jahr S, Hentze H, Englisch S, *et al*. (2001) DNA fragments in the blood plasma of cancer patients: Quantitations and evidence for their origin from apoptotic and necrotic cells. *Cancer Res* **61**: 1659–1665.

35. Murtaza M, Dawson SJ, Pogrebniak K, *et al*. (2015) Multifocal clonal evolution characterized using circulating tumour DNA in a case of metastatic breast cancer. *Nat Commun* **6**: 8760.

36. Cohen JD, Li L, Wang Y, *et al*. (2018) Detection and localization of surgically resectable cancers with a multi-analyte blood test. *Science* **359**: 926–930.

37. Hall C, Clarke L, Pal A, *et al*. (2019) A review of the role of carcinoembryonic antigen in clinical practice. *Ann Coloproctol* **35**: 294–305.

38. Blyuss O, Burnell M, Ryan A, *et al*. (2018) Comparison of longitudinal CA125 algorithms as a first-line screen for ovarian cancer in the general population. *Clin Cancer Res* **24**: 4726–4733.

39. Nash Z, Menon U. (2020) Ovarian cancer screening: Current status and future directions. *Best Pract Res Clin Obstet Gynaecol* **65**: 32–45.

40. Bronkhorst AJ, Ungerer V, Diehl F, *et al*. (2020) Towards systematic nomenclature for cell-free DNA. *Hum Genet* **40**(4): 565–578.

41. Al-Soud WA, Radstrom P. (2001) Purification and characterization of PCR-inhibitory components in blood cells. *J Clin Microbiol* **39**: 485–493.

42. Sidstedt M, Hedman J, Romsos EL, *et al*. (2018) Inhibition mechanisms of hemoglobin, immunoglobulin G, and whole blood in digital and real-time PCR. *Anal Bioanal Chem* **410**: 2569–2583.

43. Schrader C, Schielke A, Ellerbroek L, Johne R. (2012) PCR inhibitors – Occurrence, properties and removal. *J Appl Microbiol* **113**: 1014–1026.

44. Yokota M, Tatsumi N, Nathalang O, *et al*. Effects of heparin on polymerase chain reaction for blood white cells. *J Clin Lab Anal* **13**: 133–140.

Chapter 4

Maximizing Yield from Plasma Circulating DNA Extraction

Florence Mauger and Jean-François Deleuze

Abstract

Circulating cell-free DNA (cirDNA) has showed great promise as a sensitive and relevant noninvasive biomarker for liquid biopsies, but it is highly fragmented and often present in low-abundance in plasma/serum. Consequently, the extraction method needs to be very efficient to recover all fragment sizes and in particular, the short-length fragments. It is important to choose the most appropriate extraction method for each application and to optimize extraction steps to maximize the yield and the recovery of all fragment sizes of isolated cirDNA from plasma.

A number of modified phenol–chloroform protocols, column-based, and magnetic bead commercial kits have been developed and compared for isolating cirDNA from different volumes of healthy individual, cancer patient, or maternal plasma. Although, there is not a universal method for all applications, the QIAamp Circulating Nucleic Acid kit, which is the most commonly used kit, appears to be the most effective and versatile kit to maximize the yield of total and tumor-derived as well as fetal cirDNA allowing genetic analysis from a few milliliters of plasma. Epigenetic marks of cirDNA can also be analyzed and a methylation-on-beads protocol has been established to extract and bisulfite convert cirDNA; however, cirDNA for methylation analysis is typically isolated using conventional extraction methods.

Furthermore, an enrichment step may improve the analysis of fetal or methylated cirDNA. Extraction methods could be replaced by direct analysis of unpurified plasma by digital PCR or cirDNA enrichment step from a limited amount of plasma.

The cirDNA extraction method has to be very efficient, especially in the case of a limited amount of input material, and an automated extraction system is useful for clinical studies to ensure optimal reproducibility of samples.

In addition, standard operating procedures, Laboratory Information Management System, and ISO International Standards should be applied to ensure traceability, standardization of processing, and analytical reproducibility of the extraction of cirDNA.

Furthermore, the yield of extracted cirDNA can be quantified by fluorescent assay or qPCR and digital PCR using specific short-size fragments, and the presence of low- and/or high-molecular weight in extracted cirDNA can be identified by microfluidic electrophoresis or qPCR and digital PCR. A complete specific liquid biopsy workflow including collection, transport, biobanking, pre-analytical process, sample volume, extraction method, quantification method, and fragment-size analysis for each kind of plasma should be established to maximize the extraction yield and improve the analysis of low-abundance cirDNA.

Introduction

In the context of precision medicine, circulating cell-free DNA (cirDNA) shows great promise as a sensitive biomarker for disease prediction, diagnosis and prognosis, and also for monitoring the response to therapeutic treatment of cancer patients and others with complex diseases (Chapter 1). As the powerful clinical applications of cirDNA have evolved and improved, the number of protocols and commercial kits available for cirDNA isolation has increased. cirDNA in plasma/serum is present at low-abundance, and the tumor-derived cirDNA or fetal cirDNA that is most often of interest in diagnostic tests is only a small fraction of the total. The amount of cirDNA in plasma depends on a number of different biological parameters such as the age and sex of the patient, the stage and the type of cancer (for tumor-derived cirDNA), and the week of pregnancy (for fetal cirDNA). In addition, the yield of isolated cirDNA from plasma is dependent on experimental variables such as the type of liquid biopsy (Chapter 2), conditions of biobanking, pre-analytical processes (Chapters 2 and 3), and the extraction method. During the extraction process, cirDNA can be lost during binding, washing, and elution steps and, consequently, lower yields of extracted cirDNA are isolated. Various extraction methods from published protocols or commercial kits have been established to isolate cirDNA in the forms of total cirDNA, mitochondrial cirDNA, methylated cirDNA, tumor-derived cirDNA, donor-derived cirDNA, and fetal cirDNA from plasma. The extraction methods from plasma/serum should have enough efficiency and specificity to isolate all kinds of fragment sizes to improve the recovery of isolated cirDNA. The low quantity of cirDNA obtainable from clinical samples can impact downstream analytical techniques that require a minimum amount of sample to yield reliable data, and for this reason, the choice of extraction method to maximize yield can be critical to the success of a study. In this chapter, we outline the principles behind cirDNA isolation techniques, summarize the published literature comparing different commercial kits and in-house protocols, and review selected clinical studies with regard to the effect that the choice of cirDNA purification protocol has on experiment outcome.

Principles of cirDNA Extraction from Biofluids

DNA in plasma and serum is associated with protein complexes such as nucleosomes, and a proportion of this DNA is enclosed in extracellular vesicles.[1] To obtain pure DNA, the proteins must be removed by denaturation and digestion, and the DNA is extracted either by differential partitioning between aqueous and organic solvents or by selective binding to a silica-based matrix. These principles also form the basis of DNA extraction from cells and tissues; however, cirDNA presents a number of additional challenges. First, the cirDNA is heavily fragmented, occurring predominantly as ~170 bp fragments, with smaller populations with sizes in multiples of 170 bases. The size of the pieces corresponds to the length of DNA wrapped around a single nucleosome or multiple nucleosomes. The small size can have an impact on recovery and leads to low yields unless protocols are specifically configured for low-molecular-weight DNA. Second, cirDNA is very dilute, with concentrations as low as just a few ng per mL. With so little starting material, nonspecific binding to plastic ware during handling can contribute significantly to sample loss, and in matrix-based protocols, the elution volume must be kept low in order to maintain a reasonable concentration for downstream applications. There are two main approaches to the extraction of cirDNA: liquid–liquid extraction and matrix binding. We will consider each of these in turn.

Matrix Binding

Many commercially available cirDNA purification kits are based on column extraction using silica-based resin (**Fig. 1**). Binding to silica as a method of DNA purification has been applied for several decades[2,3]; however, the nature of the interaction is still

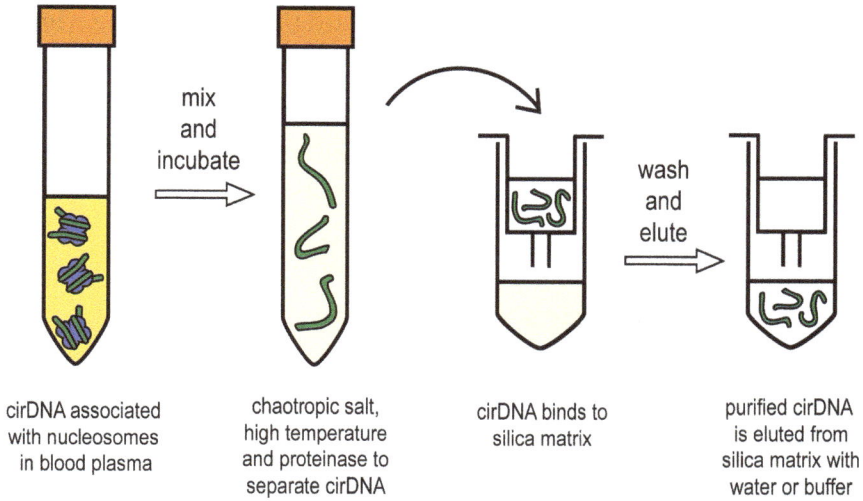

Fig. 1: Purification of cfDNA by binding to a silica matrix column. DNA is separated from nucleosomes by protease digestion at 60°C–65°C, helped by protein denaturation with detergent and chaotropic salt. Following the digestion, the DNA is captured on a silica matrix, washed, and eluted.

being elucidated.[4] Silica, with its low isoelectric point of ~pH 3, is negatively charged at neutral pH, as is DNA, creating an electrostatic repulsion. Overcoming the repulsion and binding is dependent on chaotropes that disrupt the hydrogen-bonded structure of water and appears to involve hydrophobic interactions as well as attraction between the phosphate groups in the DNA backbone and silanol.[4] The strength of the binding is influenced by multiple factors such as pH, chaotrope concentration[5,6] the size and shape of the silica particles, and the type of silanol groups on the surface.[7] Furthermore, the silica can be modified with surface molecules such as amines, metal ions, or lysine to modulate the binding affinity of different sized DNA.[8]

The advantages of matrix binding methods are that the extraction takes only a few hours, and it can be run in a high-throughput mode. Various kits have been optimized to isolate viral or genomic cirDNA from blood that is medium or high molecular weight, respectively. There are also specific extraction kits based on column or magnetic beads to isolate highly fragmented (<300 bp) cirDNA from plasma/serum.

Evaluation of Matrix Binding Protocols

As discussed earlier, many variations of matrix binding chemistry are possible, and at least 26 different methods based on matrix binding have been evaluated for cirDNA extraction efficiency (**Tables 1** and **2**). Comparison of extraction methods was performed using different extraction protocols, different samples, and volume of input, quantification, and fragment analysis methods (**Table 1**).

The Qiagen QIAamp DNA Blood Mini (QIAamp DBM) kit, originally developed for the purification of genomic DNA from leukocytes in whole blood, was one of the earliest kits used for cirDNA extraction. As a popular and robust method of DNA extraction from whole blood, it was an obvious choice to extend its use to cirDNA extraction from plasma, and it has been used in a number of studies with clinical samples.[9,10] However, the chemistry used in the kit targets the extraction of a pure sample of high-molecular-weight genomic DNA, and it does not perform well in purifying cirDNA, which is heavily fragmented. Every study that included the QIAamp DBM kit was able to identify an alternative method that gave better yields (**Tables 1** and **2**).

The QIAamp Circulating Nucleic Acids (QIAamp CNA) kit from Qiagen was released in the market in 2009 and was first evaluated in comparison with other cirDNA extraction methods by Page and colleagues in 2013.[11] This study and all but one subsequent study (n = 8) identified the QIAamp CNA kit as the best

Table 1. Workflow of cirDNA Extraction Method Comparison from Plasma/Serum of Healthy Individual and/or Cancer Patients

Extraction method	Plasma or serum	Quantification method	Fragment analysis method	Reference
Phenol–chloroform method and QIAamp DBM kit	1 mL plasma Lung cancer and benign lung disease	qPCR assay: 135 bp of *ERV-3* gene	—	(14)
NucleoSpin and QIAamp DBM kits	200 and 240 μL plasma	Fluorescent assay qPCR assays: 135 bp of *EVR-3* gene 81 bp of *β-globin* gene	Microfluidic electrophoresis Spike-in 50,10,150, 250, and 100 bp	(13)
QIAamp DBM, QIAamp Virus, Invitrogen ChargeSwitch, and Agencourt Genfind kits	600 μL plasma and Serum Healthy individual and Small cell lung cancer	qPCR assay: 77 bp of *APP* gene	PCR assays: 272 bp of *p53* gene 512 bp of *BCl-2* gene	(32)
NaI, PCI–glycogen, and guanidine–resin methods QIAamp DBM, Invitrogen ChargeSwitch, ZR, and Puregene kits	2 mL pooled sera Colorectal cancer	Fluorescent assay qPCR assays: 115 bp of *ACTB* gene 68 bp of *CDH1* gene	Electrophoresis: 200, 400, and 500 bp bands	(16)

(Continued)

Table 1. (*Continued*)

Extraction method	Plasma or serum	Quantification method	Fragment analysis method	Reference
THP method and QIAamp DBM kit	500 µL pooled plasma and serum Healthy individual	qPCR assay: *hGAPDH* gene	Spike-in: 50 or 200 ng/mL of bcl-2 plasmid DNA, genomic DNA and 100 bp ladder	(25)
QIAamp DBM, NucleoSpin kits, and MagnaPure automated system	1 mL plasma Lung cancer, benign lung disease, esophageal cancer and non-Hodgkin lymphoma cancer	qPCR assays: 92 bp of *GAPDH* gene 101 bp of *β-globin* gene 135 bp of *ERV-3* gene	—	(17)
PC method, PC phase lock tubes method, and QIAamp MinElute Virus Spin Kit	1 mL plasma Nonsmall cell lung cancer	Fluorescent assay qPCR assays: 77, 123 and 202 bp of *SERPINA1* gene *EGFR* gene	—	(29)
Schmidt and Hufnagl's PC protocols, NucleoSpin, QIAamp DBM, and Maxwell 16LEV kits	1 mL plasma Colon cancer, breast cancer, and healthy individual	qPCR assay: 98 bp of *hTERT* gene	PCR assays: 100, 200, 300, 400, and 1000 bp	(27)

FitAmp, NucleoSpin, QIAamp DBM, and QIAamp CNA kits	1 mL plasma Pooled healthy female and metastatic breast cancer	Fluorescent assay qPCR assays: 291 bp of *GAPDH* gene 67 bp of *ACTBL2* gene 64 bp of *HPRT1* gene Spike-in: *l*/hindIII: 50, 5, 0.5, and 0.05 ng	NGS sequencing of 207 amplicons: between 111 and 187 bp	(11)
Unpurified plasma, PCI method, and QIAamp DBM kit	100 μL plasma Unpurified plasma dilution 1/40 Healthy individual and coronary heart disease	qPCR assays: 90 and 222 bp of *LIPA2* gene 88 bp of *MSTN* gene 1400 to 75 copies/ 2 μL of murine plasma	Microfluidic electrophoresis	(26)
FitAmp, NucleoSpin, QIAamp DBM, and QIAamp CNA kits	0.5 and 1 mL plasma Pooled healthy female	qPCR assays: 79 bp of *TERT* gene 64 bp of *RPPH1* gene *ALUJ* sequence 135 bp of *ERV3* gene 94 bp of *GAPDH* gene 66 bp of *NACK* gene	qPCR assays: 115 bp of *ADH* gene 461 bp of *Adhβ* gene 1448 bp of *Adhδ* gene Spike-in: Fragmented ADH plasmid 106 copies/mL plasma	(12)

(Continued)

Table 1. (*Continued*)

Extraction method	Plasma or serum	Quantification method	Fragment analysis method	Reference
CGD method and QIAamp CNA kits	20–200 μL plasma cancer	Fluorescent assay qPCR assays: *KRAS, BRAF NRAS* and *PIK3CA* genes Spike-in: 5 and 20 ng/mL, standard reference DNA	—	(36)
THP, Hufnagl, Yuan and Schmidt's PC methods QIAamp CNA, NucleoSpin, Chemagic NA, Norgen cDNA and cfDNA kits	200 to 1000 μL plasma Healthy individual, metastatic cancer (colon, pancreatic, breast and lung cancer)	Fluorescence assay qPCR assays: 55 bp of *Kpn* sequence 165 bp of *DHFRP2* sequence	qPCR assays: 67 and 180 bp of *APP* gene PCR assays: 400 and 800 bp of P53 gene	(28)
PME-free, QIAamp CNA and QIAamp DSP Virus/Pathogen kits	2 mL plasma Pooled individual Nonsmall cell lung cancer	qPCR assays: 87 bp of Rnase P gene *KRAS* gene	—	(22)
QIAamp CNA kit, Maxwell RSC and MagaPure automated systems	1 mL plasma Lung and colon cancer	Fluorescent assay Digital PCR assays: *EGFR* and *KRAS* genes	Microfluidic electrophoresis	(40)

Kits/Methods	Sample	Assays	Additional	Ref.
QIAamp CNA, PME, Maxwell RSC, EpiQuick, NEXTprep-Mag cfDNA v1 and 2 kits	0.5 mL plasma Pancreatic pathology	Fluorescent assay Digital droplet PCR of *KRAS gene*	qPCR assays: 105 and 236 bp of GAPDH gene	(37)
Unpurified plasma and QIAamp CNA kit	1-2 mL plasma Metastatic colorectal cancer	Fluorometric method Digital PCR assays: *KRAS, NRAS,* and *BRAF* genes	—	(41)
QIAamp CNA, QIAamp DBM, QIAamp Ultrasens Virus and QIASymphony DSP Virus kits	1 mL plasma Pooled healthy individual	qPCR assays: 144 bp of *cxcr4b* gene 115 and 247 bp of *Alu* sequences 105 bp of *TP53* gene	Zebrafish DNA: fragmented and intact 20 ng/mL of plasma	(21)
PIBEX method and QIAamp CNA kit	5 mL Plasma Healthy individual	qPCR assays: *TERT, RPPH1, GAPDH,* and *NAGK* genes	Microfluidic electrophoresis	(39)
PME-free, QIAamp CNA, Norgen cfDNA Mag-Bind, MagMax, Maxwell RSC, ccfDNA NeoGenestar kits	250 µL and 1 mL plasma Pooled	Multiplex Digital PCR assays: 5 short PCRs and 4 long PCRs	—	(23)

Table 2:   Summary of cirDNA Extraction Method Comparison Studies

	Method	(14)	(16)	(25)	(29)	(27)	(26)	(28)
Liquid–liquid extraction	Direct analysis of unpurified plasma						■	
	optimized phenol-chloroform method						■	▨
	Guanidine resin method		▨					
	NaI method		■					
	PCI-glycogen method		▨					
	phenol-chloroform phase lock tubes method				■			▨
	triton/heat/Phenol-Chloroform method				■		▨	▨
	phenol chloroform method	■			▨	▨		▨
Matrix-based extraction	PIBEX method							
	ccfDNA NeoGeneStar kit							
	Mag-Bind cDNA kit							
	MagMAX cfDNA kit							
	NEXTprep-Mag cfDNA v2 kit							
	NEXTprep-Mag cfDNA v1 kit							
	Epiquick ccfDNA kit							
	Maxwell RSC automated system							
	BSCI SNAP method							
	QIAamp Ultrasens Virus kit							
	Akonni TruTip kit							
	NucliSens system							
	PME-free kit							
	Norgen cfDNA kit							▨
	Norgen CDNA kit							■
	Chemagic NA kit							▨
	Promega Maxwell 16LEV kit					▨		
	ZR serum DNA kit		▨					
	Puregene kit		▨					
	CGD method							
	Agencourt Genfind kit							
	QIAamp MinElute Virus Spin kit					▨		
	MagnaPure automated system							
	FitAmp kit							
	Invitrogen ChargeSwitch kit		▨					
	QIAamp DSP virus kit							
	Nucleospin (RP and HS) kit					▨		▨
	QIAamp CNA kit						■	
	QIAamp DBM kit	▨	▨	▨		▨	▨	
Reference		(14)	(16)	(25)	(29)	(27)	(26)	(28)
		Healthy and/or cancer patient circulating DNA						

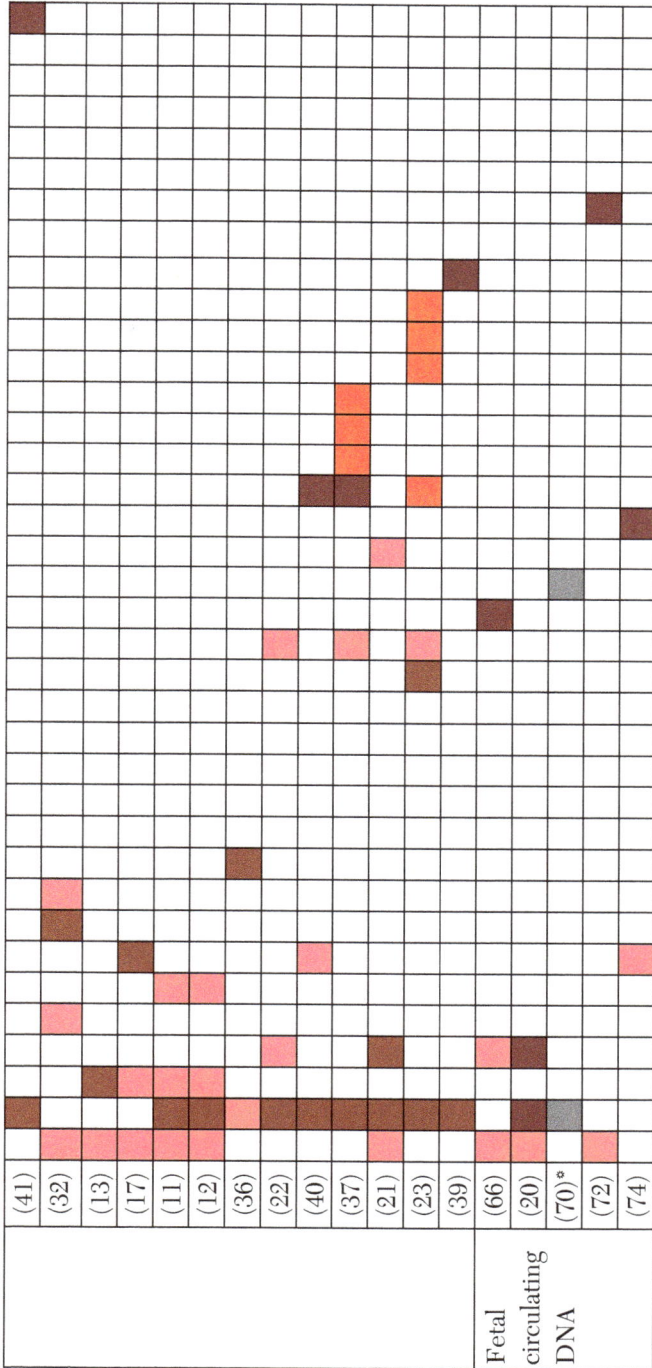

(41)
(32)
(13)
(17)
(11)
(12)
(36)
(22)
(40)
(37)
(21)
(23)
(39)
(66)
(20)
(70)*
(72)
(74)

Fetal circulating DNA

■ method was included in study

■ method gave the highest DNA yield in study

■ criteria other than total DNA yield were used to evaluate method

*Akonni TruTip method had a lower total yield of DNA but a higher percentage fraction of fetal DNA.

or joint-best-performing DNA extraction kit (**Tables 1** and **2**), largely due to improved efficiency in extracting small DNA fragments.[12] While most published studies indicate that the QIAamp CNA kit is most effective for extraction of cirDNA, there remain many gaps in the literature (**Tables 1** and **2**). Of the 26 kit-based methods evaluated, 15 have been tested in only a single study, while 6 have been tested in only 2 studies. The remaining five evaluated kits (QIAamp DBM kit, QIAamp CNA kit, Macherey-Nagel Nucleospin kit, Maxwell RSC ccfDNA Plasma (Promega), and PME-free-circulating DNA extraction (Analytik Jena)), have been tested by >2 individual studies. Individual studies comparing cirDNA extraction methods are described as follows.

Two commercial kits, the NucleoSpin plasma XS (Macherey-Nagel) kit and the QIAamp DBM kit were compared using 200 μL (Rapid protocol: RP) or 240 μL (High-sensitivity protocol: HS) of colorectal cancer plasma.[13] The recovery of cirDNA was measured using a PicoGreen assay (Invitrogen) and two qPCR assays, 135 bp of *ERV-3* gene[14] and 81 bp of *β-globin* gene, and fragment sizes were measured using the Agilent 2000 Bioanalyzer.[15] The NucleoSpin kit demonstrated a good recovery of spike-in of 50, 100, 150, 250, and 1000 bp of fragmented DNA compared to the QIAamp DBM kit, with best recovery of the 50 bp fragment. In addition, the *β-globin* assay showed PCR inhibition with the eluate input of the QIAamp DBM kit.

In another study, seven methods were compared, including a phenol–chloroform isoamyl with glycogen (PCI–glycogen), a sodium iodide method (NaI), a guanidine–resin protocol, and four commercial kits: QIAamp DBM, Invitrogen ChargeSwitch, ZR Serum DNA and Puregene DNA Purification System Cell, and Tissue kits.[16] The PCI–glycogen, NaI method, and the QIAamp DBM kit extracted higher yield of cirDNA from 2 mL of 12 pooled colorectal cancer sera quantified by a Quant-it™ dsDNA HS assay (Invitrogen). The NaI method had the highest yield measured by qPCR assays of a 68 bp *CDH1* gene and of a 115 bp *ACTB* gene. Moreover, for the NaI and PCI–glycogen methods, the size of the smallest fragments (200 bp) was also detected.

Two column-based kits, the QIAamp DBM kit, The NucleoSpin kit, and the automated MagNAPure isolation system (Roche Diagnostics) were compared using 1 mL of plasma from lung cancer, benign lung disease, esophageal cancer, and non-Hodgkin lymphoma cancer patients.[17] Extracted cirDNA was quantified using three qPCR assays of 92, 101, and 135 bp targeting the *GAPDH*, *β*-globin, and *ERV-3* genes, respectively.[14,18,19] The quantity of extracted cirDNA was between 1.6 and 2.9 ng/mL with the QIAamp DBM kit, 4.9 and 8 ng/mL for the NucleoSpin kit, and the highest yield, 12.4 and 28.1 ng/mL, was obtained for the MagNA Pure system.

Four commercial kits, the QIAamp DBM kit, the QIAamp CNA kit, the NucleoSpin kit, and the FitAmp Plasma/Serum DNA isolation (Epigentek) kit, were compared using 1 mL of pooled healthy female plasma.[11] Three qPCR assays of the *GAPDH* (291 bp), *ACTBL2* (67 bp), and *HPRT1* (64 bp) genes, and a Qubit HS dsDNA Assay (Life Technologies) were used to quantify cfDNA and showed that the two QIAamp kits (mean 264.8 ng/mL for QIAamp DBM and 239.85 ng/mL for QIAamp CNA) had a 10-fold higher yield than the two other kits. Given the results of other studies,[12,20,21] it is somewhat unexpected that the QIAamp DBM and QIAamp CNA kits recovered similar yields of cirDNA from plasma. However, the level of cirDNA in the plasma samples used was anomalously high for control plasma (~250 ng/mL), raising the possibility that in addition to low-molecular-weight cirDNA, the plasma also contained a large amount of high-molecular-weight genomic DNA, and the QIAamp DBM and CNA kits recover high-molecular-weight DNA with equal efficiency.[12,21] A spike-in of λ/*Hind*III DNA (Ambion) of 50–0.05 ng/plasma demonstrated that the QIAamp CNA kit gave the highest yield of the smallest 564-bp fragment and gave similar recovery of the 23-bp fragment compared to the QIAamp DBM kit.[11] cirDNA was then isolated from 1 mL of plasma from four metastatic breast cancer patients using the two QIAamp kits and sequenced using the Ion AmpliSeq™ Cancer Hotspot Panel v2. The recovery fragment size and sequencing coverage were similar for both kits.

Another study compared the same four kits using pooled and individual healthy female plasma.[12] cirDNA was quantified using seven qPCR assays of 79 bp of the *TERT*, 64 bp of the *RPPH1*, 135 bp of the *ERV3*, 94 bp of the *GAPDH*, 66 bp of the *NAGK* genes and *ALUJ* sequences, a commercial ValidPrime™ assay, and a digital droplet PCR. A fragmented *ADH* plasmid was spiked to samples to estimate the recovery. qPCR assays of 115 bp of *ADH*, 461 bp of A*dhβ*, and 1448 bp of A*dhδ* were used to estimate the extraction efficiency. The QIAamp CNA kit had the better efficiency (80%) for all fragment sizes and gave the best representation of smaller-size fragments (83%). The recovery efficiency, compared to the QIAamp CNA kit, was 2-fold and 4.8-fold lower for both the QIAamp DBM and the NucleoSpin kits, respectively. The QIAamp DBM kit had a better efficiency than the NucleoSpin kit, but the proportion of shorter fragments was lower than for the QIAamp CNA and the NucleoSpin kits. QIAamp kits had a good reproducibility in which the correlation variance was approximately 10% for all assays. The largest difference measured was more than 2-fold higher between the lowest *ERV3* and highest *TERT* measurements. The mean quantity of total cirDNA measured using all seven PCR assays was about 2500 copies/mL

(8 ng/mL) for individual plasma. A confidence interval of mean copy number based only on three reference genes — *TERT*, *RPPH1*, and *ERV3* could give sufficient estimation of the total cirDNA. Furthermore, these two comparison studies, which used the same four kits, showed that the QIAamp CNA kit gave a higher yield of cirDNA and it was the best method to recover short fragment lengths from 1 mL of plasma samples of healthy individuals and cancer patients.[11,12]

Three commercial kits, the PME-free-circulating DNA extraction (Analytik Jena), the QIAamp DSP Virus/Pathogen (DSP virus/Pathogen) Midi (Qiagen), and the QIAamp CNA were also compared using 2 mL plasma from pooled individual and NSCLC patients.[22] The cirDNA was quantified using the ABI TaqMan Rnase P Detection Reagent kit (87 bp), and *KRAS* mutations were analyzed using the rascreen *KRAS* RGQ kit (Qiagen). Extraction was achieved using all three kits but the QIAamp CNA gave a higher yield of cirDNA (3.03 ± 2.19 ng/μL): 3.6-fold and 5.7-fold higher than Analytic Jena's and DSP Virus/Pathogen, respectively. This study also demonstrated the necessity of standardization of pre-analytical steps such as sample collection tubes, incubation time, centrifugation steps, input of plasma, and extraction methods to improve the detection of mutations and the yield of cirDNA.

Three column-based kits, the QIAamp CNA, the Plasma/Serum Cell-free Circulating DNA Purification Midi (Norgen), and the PME-free-circulating DNA extraction, and four magnetic-bead-based kits, the Mag-Bind circulating DNA (Omega Bio-Tek), MagMAX Cell-free DNA isolation (Life Technologies), Maxwell RSC, and Circulating Cell Free DNA (NeoGeneStar), were also compared starting with 1 mL of control pooled plasma except for the Norgen and NeoGenestar kits (250 μL).[23] The yield and fragment sizes of extracted cirDNA were then analyzed by digital droplet PCR using a multiplexed assay targeting nine single-copy genomic loci, which contained five PCRs (67–75 bp) labeled with FAM and four PCRs labeled with TET ranging between 439 and 522 bp. The highest median yield (1.936 haploid genome equivalent/mL) was obtained with QIAamp CAN kit with 89% of low-molecular-weight fraction. Although, the median yield extracted from Norgen was not significantly different (1.760 copies/mL plasma, t-test p = 0.427), it was more variable; however, it was adapted to extract low input samples (250 μL). MagMax was the magnetic beads method that allowed the highest mean yield even though it was significantly lower than the QIAamp CNA kit (1.515 copies/mL) but the low-molecular-weight fraction is comparable (90%).

Finally, four QIAamp kits including the CNA, the DBM, the Ultrasens Virus, and the QIASymphony DSP Virus (QS-DSP) were compared using 1 mL of plasma pooled from healthy donors.[21] High and low molecular weights of zebrafish DNA were spiked at 20 ng/mL of plasma and quantified using qPCR assays of 144 bp targeting the *cxcr4b* gene. Three qPCR assays of 115 bp and 247 bp of Alu sequences and 105 bp of the *TP53* gene were also used. The QIAamp CNA and QS-DSP kits obtained 40% of recovery of the spike-in and have a Alu247/Alu105 ratio of about 0.1–0.15. Furthermore, the QIAamp DBM kit was more efficient in extracting high-molecular-weight DNA, and the Ultrasens Virus KIT had the lowest efficiency for both high and low molecular weights. The authors also demonstrated that the carrier RNA improved yields of cirDNA isolated from both QIAamp CNA and QS-DSP kits.

Evaluation of Phase Partitioning Protocols

Liquid–liquid extraction (also referred to as two-phase extraction or phase partitioning) is based on the partitioning of molecules between a polar aqueous phase and a nonpolar organic phase, typically phenol or a mixture of phenol and chloroform.[24] DNA is charged and will partition into the aqueous phase, while the solubility of proteins in water is dependent on polar amino acid residues facing to the outside of the folded protein. Unfolding in the presence of phenol exposes the hydrophobic amino acid side chains and the protein partitions irreversibly into the organic phase. Phenol is denser than water, so the two phases can be separated by centrifugation, and the DNA is finally collected from the aqueous phase by precipitation (**Fig. 2**). Various modifications can be introduced to improve the efficiency of the extraction process including the addition of isoamyl alcohol to the phase-partitioning mix,[16] a heat denaturation step,[25,26] and removal of bulk proteins by a salt precipitation step prior to the two-phase extraction.[14,27]

A number of studies evaluated liquid–liquid extraction protocols and compared the yield with matrix-based methods (**Tables**

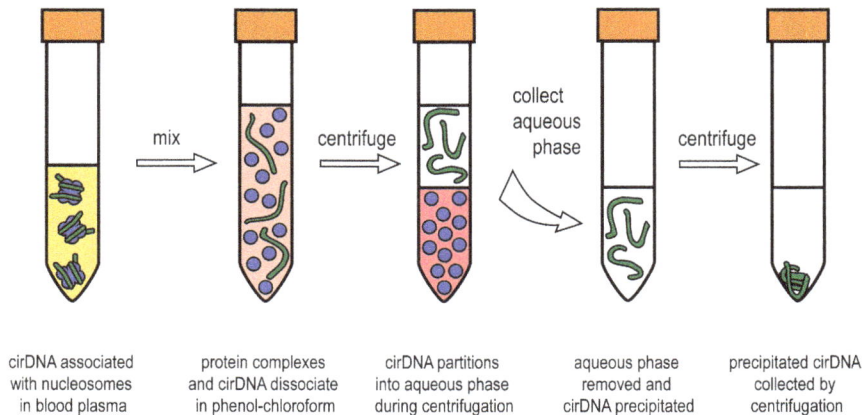

| cirDNA associated with nucleosomes in blood plasma | protein complexes and cirDNA dissociate in phenol-chloroform | cirDNA partitions into aqueous phase during centrifugation | aqueous phase removed and cirDNA precipitated | precipitated cirDNA collected by centrifugation |

Fig. 2: Two-phase extraction to purify cfDNA from plasma. The plasma sample is agitated with a phenol–chloroform mixture to unfold proteins and dissociate the cfDNA from nucleosomes. The cfDNA partitions into the aqueous phase, which is separated from the organic phase by centrifugation. The cfDNA is collected from the aqueous phase by precipitation.

1 and **2**). All but one found that the liquid–liquid extraction method gave a greater DNA yield than any commercial kit; however, there are two reasons why this does not necessarily mean that phase partitioning is generally more efficient than matrix binding for the purification of cirDNA. First, there may be an element of publication bias in the tendency to publish in-house phenol–chloroform extraction methods that perform better than established commercial protocols but not vice-versa (i.e., the observation that an in-house phenol–chloroform extraction performs worse than a commercial kit is not likely to be written up for publication). Second, and more importantly, only a single study compared phase-partitioning methods against the best performing of the matrix binding kits (QIAamp CNA kit), and this study found that better yield was obtained with the QIAamp CNA kit, as well as the Norgen Plasma/serum Circulating DNA Purification Mini kit[28]. Hence, while it would be fair to say that two-phase extraction is a better choice than the extensively evaluated QIAamp DBM kit, two-phase extraction has not been extensively tested against the best-performing matrix binding methods (**Tables 1** and **2**). Individual studies of phase-partitioning methods are summarized in **Tables 1** and **2** and are discussed as follows.

A modified salting-out method was established by Schmidt *et al.*, using 1 mL of plasma and compared to the QIAamp DBM Kit.[14] The cirDNA was quantified using qPCR assay of 135 bp of the *ERV-3* gene. The mean yield of cirDNA was 7.8 and 4 ng/mL from lung cancer patients and 15.8 and 3 ng/mL for benign lung disease patients extracted by Schmidt's protocol and the QIAamp DBM kit, respectively. Thus, this protocol allowed up to a 5-fold higher yield of cirDNA compared to the QIAamp DBM kit.

The mentioned protocol[14] was further refined by Hufnagl *et al.*[27] by eliminating one of the DNA precipitation steps and using a slightly different salt concentration. It was compared to the Maxwell 16 LEV DNA purification kit (Promega), the QIAamp DBM kit, the NucleoSpin kit, and Schmidt's protocol[14] using 1 mL of plasma from healthy individuals and colon and breast cancer patients. The cirDNA was quantified using a qPCR assay of 98 bp of the *hTERT* gene. Both published phenol–chloroform protocols gave a higher yield of cirDNA than the commercial kits, but Hufnagl's protocol[27] gave a 4-fold higher yield (86.91 and 755.4 pg/μL for 1 mL of healthy and colon cancer patients, respectively) compared to Schmidt's protocol. The authors speculated that reducing the DNA precipitation steps avoided some loss of DNA. Integrity of cirDNA was evaluated using PCR products of 100, 200, 300, 400, and 600 bp.[30] These fragments were detected using all extraction methods and the cirDNA from cancer patients was found to be more fragmented compared to healthy patients. Mutation detections of *KRAS* codon 12–13 or *BRAF* V600E showed an increase of the amount of cirDNA in cancer patients compared to healthy plasma.

A Triton/Heat/Phenol–chloroform protocol (THP) was developed by Xue *et al.*[25] It was compared to the QIAamp DBM kit using 500 μL of pooled healthy plasma or serum spiked with 50 or 200 ng/ml of bcl-2 plasmid DNA or genomic DNA and Quick-Load (New England Biolabs) 100 bp DNA ladder. The mean yields of cirDNA, quantified using the *hGAPDH* qPCR assay,[31] were 4.73 ng/ml and 1.67 ng/mL for the THP protocol and the QIAamp DBM kit, respectively. The efficiency of the THP method was higher (38.7%) compared to the QIAamp DBM kit (18.6%).

Yuan *et al.* evaluated the improvement in yield gained by using phase-lock tubes to isolate cirDNA from 1 mL of nonsmall-cell-lung cancer (NSCLC) patient plasma.[29] The tubes contain a gel that remains between the aqueous and the organic phase following centrifugation and enables easy collection of the aqueous phase. The tubes were compared to both the conventional phenol–chloroform protocol and the QIAamp MinElute Virus Spin Kit (Qiagen). The quantity of cirDNA was then measured using three qPCR assays of 77, 123, and 202 bp of the *SERPINA1* gene and a NanoDrop Spectrometer. The efficiency of the extraction method was also evaluated by mutation detection of exon 9 of the *EGFR* gene using both mutant-enriched PCR coupled with Sanger sequencing and the DxS *EGFR* mutation test kit (DxS LtD). The phase-lock tubes allowed extraction of a higher yield of cirDNA compared to the standard PCR protocol. The amount of extracted cirDNA using this modified protocol was about 20% higher, and the proportion of long fragments (>202 bp) was significantly higher (54.2%) compared to the QIAamp Virus kit (32.2%). In addition, both the detection of mutant *EGFR* and the quantity of tumor-derived cirDNA were higher with this protocol.

Finally, Mauger *et al.* compared 11 different methods including 5 liquid–liquid extractions and 6 matrix-based methods, quantitating the yield by qPCR.[28] The protocol described by Hufnagl *et al.*[27] was identified as the most efficient of the phase-partitioning extractions but overall less effective than the QIAamp CNA kit or the cfDNA kit from Norgen.[28] There was large variation in the performance of the different methods on different sample types, for example, cancer versus control, possibly reflecting differences in the size distribution of the DNA in the samples. This was the only study to include Qiagen's CNA kit in comparisons with two-phase extractions.

Liquid–liquid extraction protocols have several advantages: they are relatively inexpensive compared with column-binding kits, and they give more control over plasma input volume and final sample volume allowing greater flexibility in concentrating the DNA sample. The disadvantages are that they are time con-suming, taking up to 2 days, and involve considerable handling of noxious reagents such as phenol.

Samples with Special Volume Requirements

Some protocols lend themselves better to small or large volumes of plasma. Where the plasma volume is very small, disproportion-ate DNA losses can occur through nonspecific binding to plastic during handling, and the protocol must be compatible with a very low elution or resuspension volume in order to minimize sample dilution. Conversely, large volumes of plasma require specialized plastic ware in order to accommodate sufficient sample volume to avoid an unmanageable number of pipetting steps.

CirDNA Extraction from Low Plasma Volume Input

In the case of low input of plasma/serum, it is crucial to use the most efficient extraction method to maximize the yield of isolated cirDNA from a limited amount of sample. Several studies com-pared extraction methods starting from small volumes of plasma (**Tables 1** and **2**).

Four commercially available kits (QIAamp DBM, QIAamp MiniElute Virus Spin, Agencourt Genfind Blood and Serum Genomic DNA Isolation (Agencourt), and Invitrogen Charge-Switch), were compared using 600 μL of plasma and serum from healthy and small cell lung cancer (SCLC) patients.[32] The quantity of extracted cirDNA was measured using a 77-bp qPCR assay of the *AAT* gene. The QIAamp Virus kit gave the highest yield of cirDNA, and the cirDNA in SCLC patients was higher compared to the healthy individuals in plasma (24.5 and 5.1 ng/mL, respec-tively); however, there was no significant difference between patients and controls in serum. The fragment size of the extracted DNA was estimated using PCR of the *p53* gene (272 bp) and the *BCl-2 gene* (512 bp). The ratio of 272/77 bp fragments was higher in SCLC patients compared to healthy controls (13% and 8%, respectively), and the 512 bp fragment was not detected in the healthy plasma samples. In addition, this study showed that the plasma was more reliable than serum analysis of tumor-derived cirDNA.

Another study used plasma to compare cirDNA extraction from 11 methods and establish a complete workflow to isolate, quantify, and characterize cirDNA isolated from small sample volumes (as little as 200 μL).[28] Five published protocols[14,25,27,29] — THP, Hufnagl, Yuan and Schmidt's PC, and five kits — QIAamp CNA, NucleoSpin (HS and R protocols), the Chemagic NA extraction (Perkin-Elmer), and both Norgen Plasma/Serum Circulating DNA Purification Mini (Norgen cDNA) and cell-free Circulating DNA Purification Mini (Norgen cfDNA), were compared using 10 plasma samples from metastatic cancer patients (colon, pancreatic, lung, and breast) or healthy individuals. The cirDNA was quantified by Qubit HS dsDNA Assay (Life Technologies) and two qPCR assays using a standard curve of fragmented genomic DNA. The qPCR assays targeted a repetitive sequence throughout the genome, *Kpn* (55 bp), and a microsatellite sequence, *DHFRP2* (165 bp). NucleoSpin, QIAamp CNA, both of the Norgen kits and the two modified PC protocols[27,29] were found to be suitable for small volumes of plasma. Moreover, for the protocols that gave higher amounts of cirDNA, all quantification methods gave similar results. The Norgen cDNA and QIAamp CNA kits showed the best accuracy and reproducibility. Previously, qPCR assays of the *APP* gene (67 and 180 bp)[33,34] and qPCRs (400 and 800 bp) of the *p53* gene[35] showed that there was no bias of small-size fragments for the Norgen cDNA and QIAamp CNA kits. The Norgen cDNA kit allowed extraction of the highest amount of cirDNA from a small amount of plasma.

A new technology based on a proprietary, undisclosed enrichment and recovery of cirDNA from droplet volumes of plasma (CGD method) was reported by Spurgin and colleagues.[36] CGD extraction from 20 to 200 μL of cancer plasma was compared to the QIAamp CNA kit. The cirDNA obtained was quantified by Qubit HS and BR assays and by qPCR assays of *KRAS*, *BRAF*, *PIK3CA*, and *NRAS* genes. The average yield of cirDNA was an astonishing 92.5 ng per μL of plasma for the CGD enrichment method compared to 0.42 ng per μL of plasma for the QIAamp CNA kit, even though the plasma input was 10-fold lower compared to QIAamp CNA kit. The CGD method yielded size distributions from 100 to 500 bp. Furthermore, the comparison of Ct values of qPCR assays showed that this protocol recovered at least 100-fold more amplifiable DNA than the QIAamp CNA kit. Spike-in of 5 ng/mL of standard 4 Reference DNA and 20 ng/mL of standard 6 Reference DNA (Horizon Dx) showed 6/10 and 12/20 mutations detected in cirDNA extracted from CGD method and no mutations were detected in cirDNA isolated from the QIAamp CNA kit. Finally, the sequencing analysis showed that the quality, the quantity of the reads, and the detection of mutations were higher for this enrichment technology compared to the QIAamp CNA kit.

Finally, QIAamp CNA, PME-free-circulating DNA extraction, and magnetic beads methods (including the Maxwell RSC ccfDNA (Promega), the EpiQuick Circulating Cell-Free DNA Isolation (Epigentek) and two consecutive versions of the NEXTprep-Mag cfDNA Isolation kit (Bioscientific)) were compared using 0.5 mL of plasma. Ten plasma samples were analyzed, including five from patients with *KRAS* mutations related to pancreatic pathology.[37] Digital droplet PCR was used to quantify total cirDNA and *KRAS* mutations. cirDNA integrity measurement was performed by qPCR using two amplicons of 105 and 236 bp targeting the *GAPDH* gene and the Qubit assay was used to quantify cirDNA. QIAamp CNA and Maxwell RSC allowed similar average yields of 56.49 and 62.57 copies/µL, respectively, and detection of *KRAS* mutations. Whereas the PME and the NEXTprep-Mag (version 2) kits enabled less yields of 4.06 and 6.08 copies/µL, respectively. CirDNA extracted from EpiQuick and NEXTprep version 1 cannot be amplified by digital droplet PCR due to the presence of inhibitors. qPCR analysis of both amplicons showed that QIAamp CNA and Maxwell RSC were similar, whereas efficiency of the other kits for isolation of short fragments were lower.

cirDNA Extraction from High Plasma Volume Input

Given the low concentration of cirDNA in plasma, one approach to increasing yield where sufficient sample volume is available is to simply start with a higher input of plasma into the extraction protocol. However, the plastics supplied with commercial kits may not easily accommodate sample input volumes above 1 or 2 mL. The QIAamp CNA kit is designed to process up to 5 mL of sample, and a single study has shown linear recovery of endogenous cirDNA up to 17.5 mL of plasma input, with no column blockage.[38] In this context, one advantage of liquid–liquid extraction protocols is that they scale up easily, and the purified cirDNA is recovered at the final step by resuspension of a precipitated pellet, allowing manyfold concentration of the sample. In contrast, column-based methods may require several consecutive elutions from the membrane to maximally recover the cirDNA, leading to some sample dilution.

An alternative extraction method called Pressure and Immiscibility-Based Extraction (PIBEX) that is centrifugation-free has been developed and compared with the most commonly used QIAamp CNA kit using 5 mL of plasma samples of seven healthy individuals.[39] The PIBEX method takes advantage of a polarity difference between liquids for a vacuum-driven flow system to operate under a low vacuum pressure throughout the entire process. The total cirDNA concentration was quantified by qPCR using *TERT*, *RPPH1*, *GAPDH*, and *NAGK* genes. The concentration of extracted cirDNA from both methods was between 1.8 and 44 ng/mL and the efficiency of the PIBEX method was higher than the QIAMP CNA kit for three genes except for *RPPH1* qPCR. The size of cirDNA was also compared using microfluidic electrophoresis (Bioanalyzer 2100, Agilent) and showed peaks at 169 and 172 bp for PIBEX method and QIAMP CNA kit, respectively.

cirDNA Extraction by Automated Systems

cirDNA extraction from plasma/serum can be performed using commercially available automated systems that are based on magnetic bead isolation. Maxwell RSC automated systems showed similar isolation efficiency from 0.5 mL of plasma but less efficiency from 1 mL of plasma compared to the QIAamp CNA kit.[23,37] The MagNAPure automated system had 2–3-fold higher efficiency than the NucleoSpin kit and 5–10-fold higher efficiency than the QIAamp DBM kit.[17]

Another study compared these automated systems with the most effective QIAamp CNA kit.[40] cirDNA was extracted from 1 mL of plasma from lung and colon cancer patients followed by quantification using Qubit fluorometer and fragment length analysis by the Agilent 2100 Bioanalyzer prior to digital PCR quantification of mutations. The median concentration of cirDNA of 33 plasma samples was 1.25 ng/µL and 1.08 ng/µL per plasma from Maxwell RSC system and QIAamp CNA kit, respectively. cirDNA extraction of 26 plasma samples using both automated systems showed that MagNAPure system extracted significantly less cirDNA yield than Maxwell RSC. 88 % of cirDNA extracted from automated systems showed nucleosome-bound DNA such as mono-, di-, tri- nucleosomes and long-fragment cirDNA. The recovery of fragments, between 150 and 200 bp, was higher for MagNAPure compared to Maxwell RSC systems. In addition, there was not a significant difference in the quantification of *EGFR* and *KRAS* mutations according to extraction methods.

Direct Analysis of cirDNA from Unpurified Plasma

Direct analysis of plasma samples without any prior extraction method or enrichment method may be used to improve the analysis of cirDNA from a limited amount of plasma (**Tables 1** and **2**); however, this method does not lend itself to downstream applications in which purified cirDNA is required.

A strategy using direct analysis of cirDNA without prior extraction was compared to conventional cirDNA extraction methods including the QIAamp DBM kit and the Triton/Heat PCI-based method using plasma from patients with coronary heart disease and healthy plasma.[26] The unpurified plasma was diluted 1:40 with water and 6.4 µL was divided between three PCR reactions with a total volume of 48 µL, resulting in 0.05 µL final plasma volume per PCR reaction. The quantity of cirDNA was measured using 90 and 222 bp qPCR assays of the *L1PA2* gene and an 88 bp PCR assay of the *MSTN* gene. The quantity of cirDNA of untreated plasma was 2.79-fold higher than the quantity of cirDNA extracted using the QIAamp DBM kit. The flow-through of QIAamp DBM kit contained 36.7% of the total cirDNA from plasma. The liquid–liquid extraction-based method performed well only with high concentrations of cirDNA in which 87.4% of the amount of cirDNA was extracted. The analysis of distribution size from 35 to 1500 bp using a Fragment Analyzer (Advanced Analytical) showed different fragment lengths for both extraction methods depending on the sample, but analysis of cirDNA extracted from the QIAamp DBM kit showed an abundant peak around 170 bp. The direct quantification of cirDNA from unpurified plasma using qPCR assay of the *L1PA2* gene showed that cirDNA from coronary heart disease patients (20.1 ± 23.8 ng/mL) was 2-fold higher compared to healthy individuals (9.7 ± 4.2 ng/mL).

Another study compared the mutation detection of *KRAS*, *NRAS*, and *BRAF* using digital PCR in cirDNA from unpurified plasma and extracted from the QIAamp CNA kit of 17 metastatic colorectal cancer patients corresponding to 43 blood samples.[41] cirDNA was extracted from 1 to 2 mL of plasma and quantified using a fluorimetric method. A pre-amplification step is added prior to digital PCR to obtain 200–2000 copies/µL of cirDNA to perform digital PCR analysis. The detection rate was 93% in extracted cirDNA and 88% in unpurified cirDNA and the concordance rate between both groups was 91%. The mean value of mutant allelic frequency was 16.9 ±18.9 for extracted cirDNA and 18.5 ± 18.9 for unpurified cirDNA and discordant cases have under 0.5% of mutant allelic frequency. The correlation coefficient r^2 of mutant allelic frequency between both groups was 0.82.

Together, the various comparisons of extraction methods, which evaluated different input volumes and various sources of plasma/serum, using different methods of quantification or fragment analysis (**Table 1**), showed that the extraction method with the highest yield had a better efficiency in extracting shorter fragment lengths (**Table 2**). In addition, in four comparison studies, the QIAamp CNA kit was the most efficient extraction method both in yield and fragment size starting with mL volumes of plasma from healthy individuals or patients.[11,12,22,28] For limited input of plasma, extraction methods could be also replaced by enrichment methods or direct analysis of unpurified plasma to improve the analysis of cirDNA.

Recovery of Shorter Fragment Lengths from Plasma

Next-Generation Sequencing (NGS) has provided an opportunity for the investigation of various fragment lengths of cirDNA through direct sequencing. For example, mitochondrial, microbial, and tumor-derived cirDNA are differently fragmented and shorter in length when compared to nuclear cirDNA.[42]

Jiang *et al.* studied the size distribution of cirDNA fragments using the QIAamp DSP Blood (QIAamp DSP Blood) Mini Kit (Qiagen) to extract cirDNA from 3 to 4.8 mL of plasma from heptacellular carcinoma and chronic hepatitis B patients (with or without cirrhosis) and healthy individuals prior to NGS sequencing.[43] They showed that the nuclear cirDNA had a strong peak at 166 bp, mitochondrial cirDNA was shorter than the nuclear cirDNA, and tumor-derived cirDNA was shorter than nontumor-derived cirDNA.

Burnham *et al.*, used the QIAamp CNA kit to extract cirDNA from plasma of lung transplant recipients followed by a single-stranded DNA library preparation to analyze different cirDNA fragment sizes.[44] There was higher yield of fragments <100 bp for microbial cirDNA, mitochondrial cirDNA, and fragments between

160 and 166 bp for nuclear cirDNA. The size of donor-specific mitochondrial cirDNA was shorter than recipient mitochondrial donors.

Efficient extraction methods of short fragment lengths coupled with the improvement of analytical methods for short fragment length analysis or NGS sequencing allowed cirDNA detection including tumor-derived cirDNA, mitochondrial cirDNA, microbial cirDNA, and nuclear cirDNA.

Tumor-Derived cirDNA from Total cirDNA

The tumor-derived cirDNA extracted from cancer plasma represents only a small fraction of the total cirDNA (e.g. 0.01%–1.7% for colorectal cancer).[45] As such, both the extraction method and the quantification method should focus on fragment length to specifically detect tumor-derived cirDNA from total cirDNA for optimal detection of low mutations in tumor-derived ccfDNA. In describing the following studies, we note that where a purification method that doesn't efficiently capture, short cirDNA fragments was used; the results achieved likely underestimate the sensitivity of the target assay.

Diehl *et al.* have established an approach to detect and quantify the tumor-derived cirDNA from total cirDNA extracted from plasma.[46] QIAamp MinElute Virus vacuum kit (Qiagen) was used to extract cirDNA from 2 mL of plasma from patients with colorectal cancer during therapy (before surgery). Although the performance of this kit has never been compared against the QIAamp CNA kit (**Tables 1** and **2**), it has been compared against the QIAamp DNA Blood Mini Kit,[32] and the fold improvement in yield suggests that it does purify the fragmented cirDNA fraction with good efficiency. The total cirDNA was quantified using qPCR assay of the *LINE-1* gene and the ratio of mutant to wild type was measured using the BEAMing (Beads Emulsion Amplification Magnetics) assay to determine the number of tumor-derived molecules per mL of plasma. The median number of total cirDNA fragments was 4000 per mL of plasma, the median percentage of mutant cirDNA was 0.18%, and the median number of tumor-derived cirDNA fragments was 39 per mL of plasma.

In a different study, total and tumor-derived cirDNA was extracted from 500 μL of plasma from melanoma cancer patients and healthy individuals using the QIAamp DSP Virus Kit and quantified using qPCR assays of 67, 180, 306, and 476 bp.[33] Three integrity indexes (180/67, 306/67, and 476/67) were calculated, with the 67-bp fragment assumed to represent the total cirDNA. Reflecting a different cirDNA size distribution between cancer patients and healthy controls, the integrity indexes were also different, with the 180/67 ratio best at distinguishing the two populations. The proportion of 180–306-bp fragments was higher for melanoma cancer patients and the fraction of 67–180-bp fragments was higher for healthy individuals.

The QIAamp DBM kit was used to extract total and tumor-derived cirDNA from 200 μL of plasma from metastatic colorectal cancer patients and healthy individuals.[47] Fragmentation of cirDNA was estimated using qPCR assays of 60, 73, 101, 145, 185, 249, 300, 357, and 409 bp of intron 2 of the *KRAS* gene when using the same reverse primer. The quantification was optimal for the smaller 60–100-bp fragments. The concentration and fragmentation of tumor-derived cirDNA were correlated with tumor weight, and tumor-derived cirDNA had a higher fragmentation pattern. The metastatic colorectal patients had a 5-fold higher mean of cirDNA fragmentation compared to the healthy individuals. The investigators then established an allele-specific blocker qPCR assay of *KRAS* and *BRAF* genes, based on small fragments, for the simultaneous quantification of total cirDNA, the analysis of the mutant allele and the determination of the integrity index.[48] The results confirmed that cirDNA is highly fragmented and they estimated that 80% of cirDNA fragments are below 145 bp in colorectal cancer patients.

Andersen *et al.* established a *KRAS* allele refractory muta-tion system qPCR of short amplicon assay to analyze tumor-derived cirDNA extracted using the QIAamp Virus/Pathogen midi kit (Qiagen) from 2 mL of metastatic colorectal adenocarcinoma plasma.[49] The detection of *KRAS* mutation was compared using short amplicon (85 bp) and long amplicon (120 bp) assays. *KRAS* mutation is detected in 74% of samples using the short ampli-con assay and in 61% of samples using long the amplicon assay. The quantity of tumor-derived cirDNA was 3-fold higher in short compared to long amplicons. Consequently, the analysis of tumor-derived cirDNA was improved using short-fragment qPCR assays (Chapter 5).

Finally, analysis of mutant allele frequency in tumor-derived cirDNA using digital PCR assays showed no significant difference between the QIAamp CNA kit, the MagNAPure, and Maxwell RSC automated systems, and also between the QIAamp CNA kit and direct analysis of unpurified plasma obtained a correlation coeffi-cient of 0.82 for mutant allele frequencies above 0.5%.[40,41] In addi-tion, the quantification comparison of *KRAS* mutations in cirDNA, isolated using the QIAamp CNA kit, from metastatic colorectal cancer plasma samples by two digital quantification approaches and an E-*ice*-COLD-PCR enrichment method, showed the same range and concordance of mutation levels below the clinically rel-evant threshold.[50]

Epigenetic Analysis of cirDNA from Plasma

Beyond classic genetic analysis, the epigenetic profile of cirDNA, including nucleosome signature and methylation analysis, can also be analyzed. Indeed, cirDNA maintains epigenetic signatures whose characterization allows for the identification of the cellular origin of the extracted fragments, thus further expanding the value of cirDNA as a relevant biomarker beyond genetic analysis. For example, the QIAamp DBM kit was used to extract cirDNA from plasma of donors and breast cancer patients followed by NGS sequencing to analyze the nucleosome signature.[51]

Methylated cirDNA from Plasma

Conventional extraction kits are used to extract total cirDNA prior to cirDNA methylation analysis using NGS bisulfite sequencing. For example, the QIAamp DNA Micro kit (Qiagen) was used to extract 1 mL of pooled metastatic breast cancer plasma samples prior to whole-genome sequencing or targeted bisulfite amplicon sequencing.[52] The QIAamp DBM kit extracted cirDNA from hepatocellular carcinoma plasma samples before bisulfite conversion and a methylated CpG tandem amplification and sequencing method.[53] The QIAamp DSP Blood kit also isolated cirDNA from maternal plasma[54,55] and from systemic lupus erythematosus patients in fractions of IgG-bound or unbound plasma samples before bisulfite sequencing.[56] The QIAamp CNA kit has been used to extract cirDNA from 2 mL of plasma or 1 mL of serum prior to whole-genome bisulfite sequencing.[57] The QIAamp CNA protocol was optimized using the following modifications: additional wash, the elution buffer was heated at 40°C, and the elution was performed in two steps. The average concentration of cirDNA was 17.7 ± 10.9 ng/ml of plasma from healthy individuals, 49.5 ± 55.2

of plasma from lung cancer patients and 565.3 ± 1173.6 ng/ml of serum from pancreatic neuroendocrine tumor patients. Fragment sizes of cirDNA were analyzed using the Agilent 2100 Bioanalyzer, which showed, for some samples, contamination with high-molecular-weight DNA of about 10,380 bp in length. An additional step was performed to purify cirDNA using two size selections of bead purifications: 0.5 X followed by 1.6 X.

While standard DNA extraction kits have been used to extract methylated cirDNA as part of the total cirDNA pool, a specific extraction method has also established for cirDNA methylation analysis. Keeley *et al.* developed a methylation-on-beads (MOB) protocol that used silica superparamagnetic beads to extract and bisulfite convert cirDNA from large volumes (up to 2 mL) of plasma or serum.[58] It was compared to the conventional phenol–chloroform method and the QIAamp CNA kit using a qPCR assay of the *β-actin* gene to quantify methylated cirDNA. The extraction efficiency of the MOB protocol was 1.5–5-fold higher compared to the PC protocol and the QIAamp CNA kit and the sensitivity was improved by 25-fold.

Another strategy for methylated cirDNA analysis is the extraction of total cirDNA from plasma followed by an enrichment step for methylated fragments prior to NGS sequencing. A methyl-binding protein capture protocol (MBD-cap) used the QIAamp CNA kit to extract cirDNA from 35 mL of plasma followed by a MethylMiner kit (Invitrogen) to isolate methylated cirDNA prior to a modified version of ChiP-Seq Illumina NGS sequencing.[38] The total cirDNA was 6.9–10.7 ng/mL of plasma. The enrichment using the methyl binding MBD2 of methylated cirDNA allowed 10.2%–14.9% of recovery and a fragment size around 180 bp. Finally, a whole-genome sequencing method used the QIAamp CNA kit followed by methyl-CpG immunoprecipitation EpiMark

(New England Biolabs) for the isolation of methylated cirDNA from pregnant and nonpregnant patient plasma samples.[59]

Fetal cirDNA from Maternal Plasma

DNA purification methods are also used to extract fetal cirDNA from maternal plasma for noninvasive pre-natal diagnosis testing. The fetal cirDNA is present in low abundance in maternal plasma, especially in the beginning of the pregnancy, and it must represent a sufficient fraction of the total cirDNA for analysis to be successful.

Fragment Lengths from Maternal Plasma

The main challenge of extraction methods is the efficiency in extracting different sizes of fragments, especially in the case of maternal plasma. As with the tumor DNA studies described earlier, we note that extraction kits not configured for cirDNA purification would have underestimated the fragmentation and the total concentration of the DNA.

A size distribution study by Chan *et al.*, of cirDNA extracted using QIAamp DBM kit from 2 mL of plasma from pregnant and nonpregnant individuals showed that cirDNA in pregnant samples was longer than nonpregnant samples and that the fetal cirDNA was more highly fragmented: 20% of fetal cirDNA was >193 bp and 0% >313 bp as determined using targets within the *SRY* gene.[60] The same group published another study using the QIAamp DSP Blood kit to extract 4 mL of maternal plasma at 12 weeks of gestation.[61] The NGS sequencing results showed high-abundance fragments at 166 bp for maternal cirDNA, which was reduced to 143 bp for fetal cirDNA.

The size distribution of fetal cirDNA was also compared to total cirDNA by Fan *et al.*, using the NucleoSpin Plasma F kit (Macherey-Nagel) to extract total cirDNA from 1.6–2.4 mL of maternal plasma (12th to 23rd weeks of gestation with a male foetus) followed by NGS sequencing.[62] The quantity of fetal cirDNA was 0.7–5.6 ng/mL of plasma, measured using qPCR of *DYS4* on chromosome Y. The size distribution of cirDNA showed an abundant peak at 162 bp and a low-abundance peak at 340 bp. The fraction of fetal cirDNA was higher for shorter (< 150 bp) sequences for chromosome Y.

Another study by Kimura *et al.* used QIAamp DBM kit to extract total cirDNA from 1 mL of maternal plasma samples (17th to 39th weeks of gestation).[63] Fragment sizes were evaluated using Y-STR and SRY genes (100–524 bp). The study showed that the fetal cirDNA was more highly fragmented and the mean fragment size detected were approximately 286 bp ± 28 bp.

In addition, the size distribution of cirDNA has been used to separate fetal cirDNA from isolated total cirDNA.[64] A protocol for the enrichment of fetal cirDNA was established by Ramezanzadeh *et al.*, using size separation. The GenetBio genomic DNA isolation kit was used to extract total cirDNA from 200 µL of maternal plasma (12 weeks of gestation) that was separated on an electrophoresis gel and fragments below 300 bp were extracted and purified to be used for paternal mutation detection by allele-specific qPCR assay.

Finally, size distributions in plasma and exosomes from non-pregnant and pregnant donors were compared from 0.5 mL of plasma extracted using the QIAamp CNA kit. The yield of different fragment sizes was analyzed by four digital PCR *β*-actin gene assays of 76, 135, 490, and 905 bp and by Agilent 2100 Bioanalyzer.[65] The relative concentrations of 135, 490, and 905 bp per 76 bp in plasma were 39%, 18%, and 5.6 % for nonpregnant and 34%, 14%, and 23% for pregnant women, whereas the relative concentrations in exosomes were 40%, 18%, and 3.3% for nonpregnant and 30%, 12%, and 18% for pregnant women. The size distribution in plasma showed a majority of peaks between 150 and 200 bp and also peaks between 300 and 500 bp and 1000 and 10,000 bp for pregnant donors, and a very small peak between 300 and 500 bp for nonpregnant donors. The size distribution of exosomes was 150–550 bp for nonpregnant donors and between 300 and 500 bp and between 1000 and 10,000 bp for pregnant donors. Furthermore, the analysis of nonpregnant plasma pellet showed 87%, 75%, and 68% of relative concentrations of 135, 490, and 905 bp per 76 bp, and the majority of peaks were ≥1000 bp with a very small proportion between 150 and 200 bp and 600 and 1000 bp.

Comparison of Fetal cirDNA Extraction Methods

Several studies compared different extraction methods to identify fetal cirDNA from maternal plasma (**Tables 2** and **3**). They used different methods to estimate the yield of fetal cirDNA and total cirDNA starting with different sample volumes and from various weeks of gestation (**Table 3**). Seven matrix-based extractions and one phenol–chloroform protocol have been evaluated for cirDNA extraction but only the QIAamp DBM, the QIAamp can, and the QIAamp DSP virus kits have been compared by ≥ 2 studies.

The NucliSens Magnetic Extraction system, the QIAamp DSP Virus, and the QIAamp DBM kits were compared using 500 μL (for QIAamp DSP Virus) or 800 μL (for QIAamp DBM and NucliSens) of maternal plasma samples (13th to 19th or 34th to 37th weeks of gestation) from women who were *RhD* negative

Table 3. Workflow of Fetal cirDNA Extraction Method Comparison from Maternal Plasma

Extraction method	Maternal plasma	Quantification of Fetal ccfDNA	Quantification of Total ccfDNA	Reference
NucliSens, QIAamp DSP Virus and QIAamp DBM kits	500 or 800 μL plasma 13th–19th or 34th–37th *RhD*-negative woman and *RhD*-positive fetus	qPCR assay: 93 bp of *RHD* gene	*qPCR assay of GAPDH* gene	(66)
QIAamp DSP Virus QIAamp DBM and QIAamp CNA kits	200 to 1000 μL pooled plasma 8th–21th Male fetus	qPCR assay: 84 bp of *DYS14* gene	qPCR assay of specific androgen receptor region on X chromosome	(20)
QIAamp CNA and Akonni TruTip kits	5 and 7 mL plasma Pregnant with male fetus: 5.3th–13.3th Nonpregnant with spike-in male and female fragmented DNA	Duplex qPCR assay: 84 bp of *DYS14* gene Digital PCR	Duplex qPCR assay: 81 bp of *EIF2C1* gene on 1 chromosome Digital PCR	(70)
QIAamp DBM kit and THP method	200 and 500 μL plasma Pregnant 17th–28th *RhD* positive and husband *RhD* negative Nonpregnant	qPCR assay: 90 bp of *RHD* gene	qPCR assay: 102 bp of *β-actin*	(72)
MagnaPure automated system and BCSI SNAP method	500 μL plasma 7th–39th	Single base extension of exon 10 of *RHD* gene Multiplex qPCR assay of exon 3, 4, 5 and 7 of *RHD* gene	UV-spectroscopy	(74)

while their foetus was *RhD* positive.[66] The yields of fetal and total cirDNA were estimated using qPCR assays of 93 bp of the *RHD* exon 7[67] and of the *GAPDH* gene,[68] respectively. Quantities of fetal and total cirDNA were higher using NucliSens (1.7- and 2.3-folds, respectively) and DSP Virus (1.5- and 1.3-folds, respectively) kits compared to the control QIAamp DBM kit.[66]

Another study compared three QIAamp kits (DBM, DSP Virus, and CNA) for isolation of cirDNA from pooled maternal plasma (8th to 21th week of gestation with a male foetus) using two qPCR assays of 84 bp of *DYS14* on the Y chromosome,[69] and the X chromosome-specific androgen receptor region to quantify fetal and total cirDNA, respectively.[20] Different inputs of plasma and elution volumes of the extracted cirDNA were used: 1000/100 µL for the QIAamp CNA kit, 200/200 µL or 500/50 µL for the QIAamp DBM kit, and 500/50 µL for the QIAamp DSP kit. Consistent with the data obtained using plasma from nonpregnant donors, the average yield of fetal cirDNA was considerably higher for QIAamp CNA (231.45 pg/mL) and QIAamp DSP (188.13 pg/mL) kits compared to the QIAamp DBM kit (34.26 pg/mL). For the same input of plasma and elution, the yield of fetal cirDNA was 210.22 pg/mL and 97.59 pg/mL and the average quantity of total cirDNA was 7876 and 4296 pg/mL for QIAamp DSP Virus and QIAamp DBM kits, respectively. In summary, the QIAamp CNA kit was more suitable for higher volumes of plasma and the QIAamp DSP Virus kit gave a higher yield of cirDNA for low input of plasma.

The QIAamp CNA kit was also compared to the Akonni TruTip (Akonni Biosystems) kit for 5 mL (for both kits) or 7 mL (for Akonni TruTip) of nonpregnant and pregnant (5.3 to 13.3 weeks of gestation) plasma samples.[70] The amount of fetal and total cirDNA was quantified using qPCR of a duplex of 84 bp of *DYS14* on the Y chromosome[69] and 81 bp of *EIF2C1* on chromosome 1, respectively, and ddPCR.[71] Non-pregnant plasma samples were spiked with a dilution series of male fragmented DNA between 50 and 400 bp and female fragmented DNA between 100 and 1600 bp. The recovery of fetal cirDNA was 60% and 75% using male fragmented DNA and the recovery of total cirDNA was 40.6% and 93.6% using fragmented female DNA for the Akonni TruTip and QIAamp CNA kits, respectively. Both kits were very efficient in extracting small fragments, but the Akonni TruTip preferentially enriched fetal cirDNA using a step that reduced fragments above 600 bp from total cirDNA. Consequently, the quantity of cirDNA was higher for the QIAamp CNA kit but the fetal cirDNA/total cirDNA recovery ratio was higher for the Akonni TruTip.

The QIAamp DBM kit and the THP[25] method were compared using 200 μL (QIAamp DBM kit) or 500 μL (THP method) of maternal plasma from *RhD*-negative women carrying an *RhD*-positive fetus (17th to 28th weeks of gestation), and non-pregnant women (*RhD* positive).[72] Fetal cirDNA and total cirDNA were quantified using standard curves using two qPCR assays, 90 bp of the *RHD* gene exon 7, and 102 bp of the *β-globin* gene, respectively.[73] The yield, estimated using the Ct value of the fetal cirDNA was improved using the THP protocol (33.8 ± 1.6) compared to the QIAamp DBM kit (36.1 ± 2.47). In addition, the yield of total cirDNA was not significantly different for both methods: 32.2 and 30.9 for the QIAamp DBM kit and the THP method, respectively.

Finally, the MagnaPure automated system was compared to the binding on a glass surface BCSI SNAP™ card protocol (Blood Cell Storage Inc.) using 500 μL of maternal plasma (7th to 39th weeks of gestation).[74] The total cirDNA was quantified using UV-spectroscopy and fetal cirDNA was measured using *RHD* gene single base extension (52 SNPs) of a multiplex PCR of exons

3, 4, 5, and 7 and a qPCR of exon 10. The mean yield of total cirDNA extracted by BCSI SNAP™ card (33.8 ng/µL) was 2-fold higher compared to MagnaPure (15.7 ng/µL) and the mean fraction of fetal cirDNA was 116.2 for all samples. The fetal cirDNA extracted using BCSI SNAP™ card allowed the detection of more SNPs, especially in earlier pregnancy.

In summary, a number of circulating DNA kits have been used to extract fetal cirDNA from maternal plasma. Two of the five comparisons of cirDNA extraction methods (**Tables 2** and **3**) showed that the QIAamp CNA kit gave higher yields of fetal and total cirDNA from 1 mL or 5 mL of maternal plasma.[20,70]

Conclusions

Numerous extraction methods, either "in-house" or commercially available, have been developed to isolate cirDNA specifically from plasma and serum. The dual challenge for these methods is to both efficiently extract low-abundance cirDNA from the samples and to capture the variety of fragment lengths, especially when the input volume is limited. This is particularly the case for tumor-derived cirDNA and fetal cirDNA, which only represent a fraction of the total cirDNA, and are more fragmented in plasma.

Comparison of extraction methods has shown that protocols optimized for cirDNA give a higher yield and better recovery of short fragments (**Tables 1**, **2** and **3**). The choice of method is also dependent on the type of cirDNA to be analyzed, the scientific question asked, and sample limitations. There is not a universal extraction method to isolate all fragment lengths with the same recovery efficiency from all types of plasma samples (**Table 2**). Consequently, it is important to choose the most appropriate extraction method for each application and to optimize extraction steps (volume of plasma, volume of elution, standard to control the extraction recovery, etc.) to maximize the recovery of all fragment sizes and the yield of isolated cirDNA. The QIAamp CNA kit, which is the most commonly used method, appears to be the most effective and versatile method to maximize the yield of total, tumor-derived or fetal cirDNAs from a few mL of plasma (**Table 2**). However, all extraction methods have not been directly compared, they have not been optimized for all applications, for example, small versus large sample volumes and they have not been compared using the same sample, the same quantification method (fluorescent assay, qPCR, or digital PCR assays), or the same fragment analysis method (microfluidic electrophoresis, qPCR, and digital PCR assays) (**Tables 1** and **3**). It is likely that with ongoing research new techniques will emerge.

In addition, the analysis of cirDNA can also be enhanced using other approaches. Fetal cirDNA or methylated cirDNA can be enriched from isolated total cirDNA to improve the analysis. For a limited amount of plasma, the extraction step can be replaced by direct analysis of unpurified plasma by digital PCR or an enrichment step for cirDNA.

Moreover, it is crucial to standardize and optimize the process for each application especially for the analysis of clinical samples. To ensure traceability, standardization of processing, and analytical reproducibility, standard operating procedure, a Laboratory Information Management System, and ISO International Standards (ISO 20186-3: 2019) should be used for plasma sample analysis. A complete specific liquid biopsy workflow has to be developed incorporating collection, transport, biobanking, pre-analytical process, sample volumes, extraction method, quantification method, and analysis method for each kind of cirDNA and application (**Tables 1** and **3**). Each step of the process can impact the yield and fragment sizes recovery of isolated cirDNA and should be optimized, standardized, and automated to improve target detection especially in the case of low-abundance tumor cirDNA.

The dramatic results obtained in cancer diagnosis, prediction, and monitoring have created interest in using cirDNA in a broad variety of applications. Among these is the promise of cirDNA becoming a universal biomarker of disease through epigenetic analysis or the potential of cirDNA to more adequately capture tumor heterogeneity. This interest will undoubtedly lead to the development and/or improvement of new extraction for various types of liquid biopsies (e.g., urine, saliva plasma, cerebrospinal fluid) and NGS analysis methods in the very near future.

References

1. Thierry AR, El Messaoudi S, Gahan PB, *et al.* (2016) Origins, structures, and functions of circulating DNA in oncology. *Cancer Metastasis Rev* **35**: 347–376.
2. Marko MA, Chipperfield R, Birnboim HC. (1982) A procedure for the large-scale isolation of highly purified plasmid DNA using alkaline extraction and binding to glass powder. *Anal Biochem* **121**: 382–387.
3. Boom R, Sol CJ, Salimans MM, *et al.* (1990) Rapid and simple method for purification of nucleic acids. *J Clin Microbiol* **28**:495–503.
4. Shi B, Shin YK, Hassanali AA, Singer SJ. (2015) DNA binding to the silica surface. *J Phys Chem B* **119**: 11030–11040.
5. Melzak KA, Sherwood CS, Turner RFB, Haynes CA. (1996) Driving forces for DNA adsorption to silica in perchlorate solutions. *J Colloid Interf Sci* **181**: 635–644.
6. Romanowski G, Lorenz MG, Wackernagel W. (1991) Adsorption of plasmid DNA to mineral surfaces and protection against DNase I. *Appl Environ Microbiol* **57**: 1057–1061.

7. Tian H, Huhmer AF, Landers JP. (2000) Evaluation of silica resins for direct and efficient extraction of DNA from complex biological matrices in a miniaturized format. *Anal Biochem* **283**: 175–191.

8. Liu L, Guo Z, Huang Z, *et al.* (2016) Size-selective separation of DNA fragments by using lysine-functionalized silica particles. *Sci Rep*;**6**: 22029.

9. Feng J, Gang F, Li X, *et al.* (2013) Plasma cell-free DNA and its DNA integrity as biomarker to distinguish prostate cancer from benign prostatic hyperplasia in patients with increased serum prostate-specific antigen. *Int Urol Nephrol* **45**: 1023–1028.

10. Vinayanuwattikun C, Winayanuwattikun P, Chantranuwat P, *et al.* (2013) The impact of non-tumor-derived circulating nucleic acids implicates the prognosis of non-small cell lung cancer. *J Cancer Res Clin Oncol* **139**: 67–76.

11. Page K, Guttery DS, Zahra N, *et al.* (2013) Influence of plasma processing on recovery and analysis of circulating nucleic acids. *PloS One* **8**: e77963.

12. Devonshire AS, Whale AS, Gutteridge A, *et al.* (2014) Towards standardisation of cell-free DNA measurement in plasma: Controls for extraction efficiency, fragment size bias and quantification. *Anal Bioanal Chem* **406**: 6499–64512.

13. Kirsch C, Weickmann S, Schmidt B, Fleischhacker M. (2008) An improved method for the isolation of free-circulating plasma DNA and cell-free DNA from other body fluids. *Ann N Y Acad Sci* **1137**: 135–139.

14. Schmidt B, Weickmann S, Witt C, Fleischhacker M. (2005) Improved method for isolating cell-free DNA. *Clin Chem* **51**: 1561–1563.

15. Jung M, Klotzek S, Lewandowski M, *et al.* (2003) Changes in concentration of DNA in serum and plasma during storage of blood samples. *Clin Chem* **49**: 1028–1029.

16. Fong SL, Zhang JT, Lim CK, *et al.* (2009) Comparison of 7 methods for extracting cell-free DNA from serum samples of colorectal cancer patients. *Clin Chem* **55**: 587–589.

17. Fleischhacker M, Schmidt B, Weickmann S, *et al.* (2011) Methods for isolation of cell-free plasma DNA strongly affect DNA yield. *Clinica Chim Acta* **412**: 2085–2088.

18. Birch L, English CA, O'Donoghue K, *et al.* (2005) Accurate and robust quantification of circulating fetal and total DNA in maternal plasma from 5 to 41 weeks of gestation. *Clin Chem* **51**: 312–320.

19. Lo YM, Tein MS, Lau TK, *et al*. (1998) Quantitative analysis of fetal DNA in maternal plasma and serum: implications for noninvasive prenatal diagnosis. *Am J Hum Genet* **62**: 768–775.

20. Repiska G, Sedlackova T, Szemes T, *et al*. (2013) Selection of the optimal manual method of cell free fetal DNA isolation from maternal plasma. *Clin Chem Lab Med* **51**: 1185–1189.

21. Warton K, Graham LJ, Yuwono N, Samimi G. (2018) Comparison of 4 commercial kits for the extraction of circulating DNA from plasma. *Cancer Gen* **228**: 143–150.

22. Sherwood JL, Corcoran C, Brown H, *et al*. (2016) Optimised pre-analytical methods improve KRAS mutation detection in circulating tumour DNA (ctDNA) from patients with non-small cell lung cancer (NSCLC). *PloS One* **11**:e0150197.

23. Markus H, Contente-Cuomo T, Farooq M, *et al*. (2018) Evaluation of pre-analytical factors affecting plasma DNA analysis. *Sci Rep* **8**: 7375.

24. Sambrook MRGaJ. *Molecular Cloning: A Laboratory Manual*, Cold Spring Harbor Laboratory Press; 4th edition (June 15, 2012) New York.

25. Xue X, Teare MD, Holen I, *et al*. (2009) Optimizing the yield and utility of circulating cell-free DNA from plasma and serum. *Clinica Chim Acta* **404**: 100–104.

26. Breitbach S, Tug S, Helmig S, *et al*. (2014) Direct quantification of cell-free, circulating DNA from unpurified plasma. *PloS One* **9**: e87838.

27. Hufnagl C, Stöcher M, Moik M, *et al*. (2013) A modified Phenol-chloroform extraction method for isolating circulating cell free DNA of tumor patients. *J Nucleic Acids Invest* **4**: e1.

28. Mauger F, Dulary C, Daviaud C, *et al*. (2015) Comprehensive evaluation of methods to isolate, quantify, and characterize circulating cell-free DNA from small volumes of plasma. *Anal Bioanal Chem* **407**: 6873–6878.

29. Yuan H, Zhu ZZ, Lu Y, *et al*. (2012) A modified extraction method of circulating free DNA for epidermal growth factor receptor mutation analysis. *Yonsei Med J* **53**: 132–137.

30. van Dongen JJ, Langerak AW, Bruggemann M, *et al*. (2003) Design and standardization of PCR primers and protocols for detection of clonal immunoglobulin and T-cell receptor gene recombinations in suspect lymphoproliferations: Report of the BIOMED-2 Concerted Action BMH4-CT98-3936. *Leukemia* **17**: 2257–2317.

31. Ponchel F, Toomes C, Bransfield K, *et al.* (2003) Real-time PCR based on SYBR-Green I fluorescence: An alternative to the TaqMan assay for a relative quantification of gene rearrangements, gene amplifications and micro gene deletions. *BMC Biotechnol* **3**: 18.

32. Board RE, Williams VS, Knight L, *et al.* (2008) Isolation and extraction of circulating tumor DNA from patients with small cell lung cancer. *Ann N Y Acad Sci* **1137**: 98–107.

33. Pinzani P, Salvianti F, Zaccara S, *et al.* (2011) Circulating cell-free DNA in plasma of melanoma patients: qualitative and quantitative considerations. *Clinica Chim Acta* **412**: 2141–2145.

34. Salvianti F, Pinzani P, Verderio P, *et al.* (2012) Multiparametric analysis of cell-free DNA in melanoma patients. *PloS One* **7**: e49843.

35. Ebtsam R. Zahera MMA, Hanaa M, *et al.* (2012) Value of circulating DNA concentration and integrity as a screening test for detection of cancer in an Egyptian cohort. *Alexandria J Med* **48**: 187–196.

36. Spurgin J, Ford A, Athanasuleas J, Yeh C. (2015) Next-generation targeted sequencing of circulating cell-free DNA from droplet volumes of blood. *IJLSR* **3**: 23–29.

37. Sorber L, Zwaenepoel K, Deschoolmeester V, *et al.* (2017) A comparison of cell-free DNA isolation kits: Isolation and quantification of cell-free DNA in plasma. *J Mol Diagn* **19**: 162–168.

38. Warton K, Lin V, Navin T, *et al.* (2014) Methylation-capture and next-generation sequencing of free circulating DNA from human plasma. *BMC Genomics* **15**: 476.

39. Lee H, Na W, Park C, *et al.* (2018) Centrifugation-free extraction of circulating nucleic acids using immiscible liquid under vacuum pressure. *Sci Rep* **8**: 5467.

40. Perez-Barrios C, Nieto-Alcolado I, Torrente M, *et al.* (2016) Comparison of methods for circulating cell-free DNA isolation using blood from cancer patients: Impact on biomarker testing. *Transl Lung Cancer Res* **5**: 665–672.

41. Sefrioui D, Beaussire L, Perdrix A, *et al.* (2017) Direct circulating tumor DNA detection from unpurified plasma using a digital PCR platform. *Clin Biochem* **50**: 963–966.

42. Mouliere F, Rosenfeld N. (2015) Circulating tumor-derived DNA is shorter than somatic DNA in plasma. *Proc Natl Acad Sci U S A* **112**: 3178–3179.

43. Jiang P, Chan CW, Chan KC, *et al.* (2015) Lengthening and shortening of plasma DNA in hepatocellular carcinoma patients. *Proc Natl Acad Sci U S A* **112**: E1317–E1325.

44. Burnham P, Kim MS, Agbor-Enoh S, *et al.* (2016) Single-stranded DNA library preparation uncovers the origin and diversity of ultrashort cell-free DNA in plasma. *Sci Rep* **6**: 27859.

45. Diehl F, Li M, Dressman D, *et al.* (2005) Detection and quantification of mutations in the plasma of patients with colorectal tumors. *Proc Natl Acad Sci U S A* **102**: 16368–16373.

46. Diehl F, Schmidt K, Choti MA, *et al.* (2008) Circulating mutant DNA to assess tumor dynamics. *Nat Med* **14**: 985–990.

47. Mouliere F, Robert B, Arnau Peyrotte E, *et al.* (2011) High fragmentation characterizes tumour-derived circulating DNA. *PloS One* **6**: e23418.

48. Mouliere F, El Messaoudi S, Pang D, *et al.* Multi-marker analysis of circulating cell-free DNA toward personalized medicine for colorectal cancer. *Mol oncol* **8**: 927–941.

49. Andersen RF, Spindler KL, Brandslund I, *et al.* (2015) Improved sensitivity of circulating tumor DNA measurement using short PCR amplicons. *Clinica Chim Acta* **439**: 97–101.

50. Sefrioui D, Mauger F, Leclere L, *et al.* (2016) Comparison of the quantification of KRAS mutations by digital PCR and E-ice-COLD-PCR in circulating-cell-free DNA from metastatic colorectal cancer patients. *Clinica Chim Acta* **465**: 1–4.

51. Ulz P, Thallinger GG, Auer M, *et al.* (2016) Inferring expressed genes by whole-genome sequencing of plasma DNA. *Nat Genet* **48**(10): 1273–1278.

52. Legendre C, Gooden GC, Johnson K, *et al.* (2015) Whole-genome bisulfite sequencing of cell-free DNA identifies signature associated with metastatic breast cancer. *Clin Epigenetics* **7**: 100.

53. Wen L, Li J, Guo H, *et al.* (2015) Genome-scale detection of hypermethylated CpG islands in circulating cell-free DNA of hepatocellular carcinoma patients. *Cell Res* **25**: 1376.

54. Lun FM, Chiu RW, Sun K, *et al.* (2013) Noninvasive prenatal methylomic analysis by genomewide bisulfite sequencing of maternal plasma DNA. *Clin Chem* **59**: 1583–1594.

55. Sun K, Jiang P, Chan KC, *et al.* (2015) Plasma DNA tissue mapping by genome-wide methylation sequencing for noninvasive prenatal, cancer, and transplantation assessments. *Proc Natl Acad Sci U S A* **112**: E5503–E5512.

56. Chan RW, Jiang P, Peng X, *et al.* (2014) Plasma DNA aberrations in systemic lupus erythematosus revealed by genomic and methylomic sequencing. *Proc Natl Acad Sci U S A* **111**: E5302–E5311.

57. Maggi EC, Gravina S, Cheng H, *et al.* (2018) Development of a method to implement whole-genome bisulfite sequencing of cfDNA from cancer patients and a mouse tumor model. *Front Genet* **9**: 6.

58. Keeley B, Stark A, Pisanic TR, *et al.* (2013) Extraction and processing of circulating DNA from large sample volumes using methylation on beads for the detection of rare epigenetic events. *Clinica Chim Acta* **425**: 169–175.

59. Jensen TJ, Kim SK, Zhu Z, *et al.* (2015) Whole genome bisulfite sequencing of cell-free DNA and its cellular contributors uncovers placenta hypomethylated domains. *Genome Biol* **16**: 78.

60. Chan KC, Zhang J, Hui AB, *et al.* (2004) Size distributions of maternal and fetal DNA in maternal plasma. *Clin Chem* **50**: 88–92.

61. Lo YM, Chan KC, Sun H, *et al.* (2010) Maternal plasma DNA sequencing reveals the genome-wide genetic and mutational profile of the fetus. *Sci Transl Med* **2**: 61ra91.

62. Fan HC, Blumenfeld YJ, Chitkara U, *et al.* (2010) Analysis of the size distributions of fetal and maternal cell-free DNA by paired-end sequencing. *Clin Chem* **56**: 1279–1286.

63. Kimura M, Hara M, Itakura A, *et al.* (2011) Fragment size analysis of free fetal DNA in maternal plasma using Y-STR loci and SRY gene amplification. *Nagoya J Med Sci* **73**: 129–135.

64. Ramezanzadeh M, Salehi M, Farajzadegan Z, *et al.* (2016) Detection of paternally inherited fetal point mutations for beta-thalassemia in maternal plasma using simple fetal DNA enrichment protocol with or without whole genome amplification: An accuracy assessment. *J Matern Neonatal Med* **29**: 2645–2649.

65. Fernando MR, Jiang C, Krzyzanowski GD, Ryan WL. (2018) Analysis of human blood plasma cell-free DNA fragment size distribution using Eva-Green chemistry based droplet digital PCR assays. *Clinica Chim Acta* **483**: 39–47.

66. Clausen FB, Krog GR, Rieneck K, Dziegiel MH. (2007) Improvement in fetal DNA extraction from maternal plasma. Evaluation of the NucliSens magnetic extraction system and the QIAamp DSP virus kit in comparison with the QIAamp DNA blood mini kit. *Prenat Diagn* **27**: 6–10.

67. Clausen FB, Krog GR, Rieneck K, *et al.* (2005) Reliable test for prenatal prediction of fetal RhD type using maternal plasma from RhD negative women. *Prenat Diagn* **25**: 1040–1044.

68. Johnson KL, Dukes KA, Vidaver J, *et al.* (2004) Interlaboratory comparison of fetal male DNA detection from common maternal plasma samples by real-time PCR. *Clin Chem* **50**: 516–521.

69. Zimmermann BG, Maddocks DG, Avent ND. (2008) Quantification of circulatory fetal DNA in the plasma of pregnant women. *Methods Mol Biol* **444**: 219–229.

70. Holmberg RC, Gindlesperger A, Stokes T, *et al.* (2013) Akonni TruTip((R)) and Qiagen((R)) methods for extraction of fetal circulating DNA—Evaluation by real-time and digital PCR. *PloS One* **8**: e73068.

71. Fan HC, Blumenfeld YJ, Chitkara U, *et al.* (2008) Noninvasive diagnosis of fetal aneuploidy by shotgun sequencing DNA from maternal blood. *Proc Natl Acad Sci U S A* **105**: 16266–16271.

72. Keshavarz Z, Moezzi L, Ranjbaran R, *et al.* (2015) Evaluation of a modified DNA extraction method for isolation of cell-free fetal DNA from maternal serum. *Avicenna J Med Biotechnol* **7**: 85–88.

73. Wang XD, Wang BL, Ye SL, *et al.* (2009) Non-invasive foetal RHD genotyping via real-time PCR of foetal DNA from Chinese RhD-negative maternal plasma. *Europ J Clin Invest* **39**: 607–617.

74. Adamczyk T, Doescher A, Haydock PV, *et al.* (2015) The glass slide extraction system snap card improves non-invasive prenatal genotyping in pregnancies with antibodies. *Transfus Med Hemother* **42**: 379–384.

Chapter 5

Optimal Design of PCR Assays for Circulating DNA

Rikke F. Andersen

Abstract

Carefully considered assay design is essential for PCR-based methods used in circulating DNA (cirDNA) studies. Broadly speaking, there are three main contexts in which cirDNA is subjected to PCR amplification and analyses: (1) in order to quantitate overall cirDNA, or a particular cirDNA sequence; (2) in order to detect mutations or methylation; and (3) as part of sequencing library preparation. In addition to general considerations about primer/probe design, it is equally important to understand the nature and composition of cirDNA in order to optimize analyses. Throughout the research literature, many different approaches have been taken to amplify and quantify cirDNA. Differences in analytical methods influence results, such that studies become incomparable and this hampers the progress of promising clinical biomarkers.

Circulating Cell-Free DNA

The origin of circulating DNA (cirDNA) in blood and the mechanisms of release have been investigated but are not yet fully understood. In healthy individuals, the majority of the cirDNA is of hematopoietic origin.[1] Apoptosis appears to be the major release mechanism for cirDNA, but other mechanisms such as active release through particular or macromolecular structures also seem to play an important role.[2,3] The genome is not uniformly represented in circulation; there is an over-representation of Alu elements and an under-representation of long interspersed nuclear elements L1 and L2,[4-6] confirming that cirDNA is not randomly released but that active release is involved.

cirDNA Size

Nuclear DNA is wrapped around nucleosomes with linker regions between the nucleosome cores. The size of the DNA wrapped around histones and the linker DNA is 146 base pairs (bp) and 20 bp, respectively. Consistent with its proposed origin from apoptotic cells, most cirDNA is made up of short double-stranded fragments that are 166 bp in length, corresponding to the length of DNA cleaved between nucleosomes.[7] Although the size profile of cirDNA in healthy individuals is dominated by the peak at 166 bp, other fragment sizes are also seen. Smaller peaks are found at approximately 143 bp and at 10 bp intervals below that, corresponding to one turn of the DNA helix wrapped around the core histone.[8,9] This indicates that part of the nucleosomal DNA sequence is exposed to nucleases. Longer fragments corresponding to the length of DNA wrapped around two or three nucleosomes are also found but at much lower levels.[7]

Recent studies have demonstrated that the amount of short (<100 bp) fragments of cirDNA is probably more significant than previously thought.[10,11] There are a number of reasons why these very short fragments do not readily lend themselves to detection and analysis. First, they cannot be amplified in a PCR reaction if the amplicon is larger than the cirDNA fragment; even amplicons that are the same size or slightly smaller than the cirDNA fragments will not detect them, unless the position of the DNA breaks aligns closely with ends of the PCR target sequence. Second, they are difficult to observe on a gel or BioAnalyzer chip, as they seem to occur in a range of sizes, and hence do not produce a discrete, readily visible band. Finally, DNA fragments smaller than 100 bp are not captured by standard NGS library preparation protocols. Single-stranded NGS library preparation methods, which do not include a lower limit on the size of fragments sequenced, have revealed significantly shorter cirDNA fragments than traditional NGS methods. The periodicity of 10 bp peaks remained down to 50 bp.[10,12] Hence, PCR assays should consider the fragmented nature of cirDNA, and the population of cirDNA assayed will depend on the size of the target PCR products.

Nucleosomal Positioning and cirDNA Fragmentation Patterns

Nucleosomes are not evenly distributed along chromosomes. Positioning of nucleosomes is important for gene transcription, with active transcription start sites and upstream regions being without nucleosomes in order to provide access for transcription factors, and nucleosomes immediately adjacent to the transcription start site being phased in a regular pattern.[13–15] Nucleosome positioning needs to be considered in the design of PCR assays for cirDNA. Assays spanning the transcription start sites of active genes or the region between phased nucleosomes may not yield a product, as intact target DNA may be depleted from the cirDNA pool due to inter-nucleosomal fragmentation.

The number of nucleosomes is increased in exon regions compared to intron regions and especially at exon–intron and intron–exon boundaries.[16–18] Interestingly, the 146 bp length of DNA wrapped around a nucleosome is approximately equivalent to the length of an average exon.[19] Longer exons contain a higher number of nucleosomes phased within the exon.[17] The fragmentation of cirDNA is nonrandom and reflects the nucleosomal pattern. DNA within the nucleosomal core is protected from nucleases by the histones, whereas the linker regions are more exposed. In regions with fewer nucleosomes, DNA is more fragmented.[20,21] DNA cleavage is sequence-dependent with 10 positions on either side of the DNA cleavage site showing a consistent pattern of preference for specific nucleotides. In particular, cytosine is over-represented at the cleavage site and at positions 1 and –2.[20] The copy number of specific fragments of cirDNA may consequently depend on the nucleosomal positioning and specific sequence at a given DNA locus, which has implications for optimal assay design.

cirDNA Methylation

Methylation patterns are correlated with nucleosome positioning. DNA associated with nucleosomes is more highly methylated than flanking DNA and a 10-base periodicity in DNA methylation status is found in nucleosome-bound DNA. Exon regions are more methylated than intron regions, which is consistent with the higher number of nucleosomes in exons.[17]

Mitochondrial cirDNA

Mitochondrial DNA is also present in the circulation. The size profile of mitochondrial DNA is different from nuclear DNA, since mitochondrial DNA is not associated with histones and hence not degraded in the same way as nuclear DNA. According to a study by Jiang *et al.*[8] the amount of mitochondrial DNA is only 0.00045% of the total DNA in circulation even though several copies of the mitochondrial genome are present in cells. Mitochondrial DNA in circulation is very short (<100 bp) with a peak at 42 bp,[22] indicating that it is not protected from nucleases in the same way as nuclear DNA, and not degraded in a systematic way during apoptosis. By using a single-stranded library preparation method, Burnham *et al.* showed that a large proportion of the mitochondrial DNA is undetected by widely used methods. In this study, circulating mitochondrial DNA was found at a level of 0.002% of the total cirDNA.[10] By optimizing purification and NGS specifically for mitochondrial cirDNA, Zhang *et al.* found 0.14% mitochondrial DNA in circulation.[22]

Circulating Cell-Free DNA in Cancer

Early studies on the clinical utility of cirDNA focused on quantitative differences between healthy individuals and cancer patients. To obtain reliable and comparable results, it is important to understand the differences in cirDNA between these groups. In cancer patients, the level of cirDNA is often elevated compared to healthy individuals, but this is not always observed in patients with early-stage cancer, and hence the usage of quantitative differences to identify cancer patients is limited to patients with advanced disease. To expand the utility of liquid biopsies, qualitative differences such as tumor-specific somatic mutations, copy number variations, and methylation patterns can be analyzed. This invariably complicates the analyses. No universal tumor-specific marker has been identified and a panel of analyses is needed to cover various patient groups. Depending on the tissue, tumors display various degrees of molecular similarity. In some cancers, tumors harbor somatic mutations in hotspot regions and tumor-specific markers for many patients can be covered by only a few analyses. In other cancers, hardly any similarities are seen in mutation profiles and customized analyses would have to be developed for individual patients. Methylation analyses are based on the fact that various cancer-related genes are methylated in the tumor but not in normal tissue. These genes are specific for certain types of cancer and hence one analysis for all patients with the same type (or sub-type) of cancer can in theory be used.[23]

The level of cirDNA in healthy individuals is approximately 1000–10,000 genome equivalents per mL plasma (3.3–33 ng/mL).[24,25] In patients with localized disease, levels are often higher and in metastatic disease levels are significantly elevated in many cancers.[26] The fraction of tumor-derived DNA in circulation varies greatly between patients and can reach extremely high levels in metastatic disease (up to >90% DNA from tumor).[27] In localized disease, levels are lower with undetectable levels in 40%–50% of patients.[27]

Circulating tumor DNA is being investigated for use in diagnosis of cancer, monitoring of treatment response, detection of minimal residual disease, and prediction of recurrence and treatment resistance.[28] For all of these purposes, an extremely high level of sensitivity is needed in order for the assay to be clinically relevant. The current level of detection for the most sensitive methods is ~0.01% mutated DNA and is set by methodological limitations. This is equal to 1 mutated molecule in a background of 10,000 wild-type molecules. To reliably quantify this level, at least 3 mutated molecules in a background of 30,000 wild-type molecules must be analyzed. In many cases, however, the amount of DNA available from plasma samples is less than that and, therefore, does not allow for analyses of sufficient sensitivity.

The literature regarding the size profile of cirDNA in cancer patients has been inconsistent, although recent studies have been more in agreement. Several studies have reported that cirDNA fragments are longer in cancer patients,[29–32] while other studies have reported that cirDNA fragments are shorter.[24,33] With the advancement of NGS techniques, where the exact lengths of individual fragments can be determined, it is now clear that the majority of the cirDNA in both healthy individuals and cancer patients is 166-bp long, but that in cancer patients, a significant proportion of the tumor-derived cirDNA is shorter. It has been demonstrated that the size profile of cirDNA is shifted toward shorter fragment lengths with increasing fraction of tumor DNA in circulation.[8] Longer fragments are also found in the circulation but mainly in patients with lower fractions of tumor DNA.[8] These longer fragments have been speculated to be released during necrosis.[7] Long fragments have been observed by gel electrophoresis but have not been studied by NGS, as the most widely used sequencing methods are not designed for sequencing very long fragments. Hence, this fraction of cirDNA is awaiting investigation in more detail by alternative methods.

cirDNA in cancer patients appears to be released into circulation mainly by apoptosis, as in healthy individuals, but necrosis and active release may also play important roles.[34] The fraction of cirDNA released by different mechanisms may vary between patients depending on tumor characteristics (stage, location, size, tumor type, etc.) perhaps leading to different size profiles of the cirDNA in patients with different characteristics.

The integrity of cirDNA has been proposed as a marker of disease. It has been shown that fragments generally are shorter in patients with metastatic disease than patients with early-stage disease[35] and that variation in integrity index reflects disease dynamics.[30,36] However, the integrity of cirDNA may vary in different types of cancer, due to differences in the biology of DNA release from various tissues.

Circulating mitochondrial DNA has been suggested as a marker for diagnosis and prognosis in cancer. Mitochondrial DNA in cancer patients is found at a higher level, and the size profile in cancer patients shows that the DNA is even shorter than in healthy subjects.[8] It has been found that elevated levels of mitochondrial cirDNA in cancer patients are associated with a poor prognosis.[37–39]

As described earlier, nucleosomes are involved in determining gene expression and hence are positioned differently in different cell types/tissues, reflecting different patterns of gene activity. Because fragmentation occurs more frequently in regions without nucleosomes (i.e., in regions where gene expression is active), this opens up the possibility of determining the tissue of origin of cirDNA. The main portion of cirDNA is of hematopoietic and myeloid origin, but it has been shown that DNA from other tissues can be identified in circulation, corresponding to cancer tissue in a specific individual.[12] This could potentially be used to classify cancers of unknown origin, but it also offers potential for more exact and specific quantification of tumor DNA in patients with known cancers. If PCR assays are positioned at regions that are less fragmented in tumor-specific DNA than in normal DNA, a tumor-specific signal change in cirDNA concentration would be measured. This, however, requires very detailed knowledge of the fragmentation patterns of specific tissues and of nucleosome patterns in healthy and diseased individuals.

A similar concept has been demonstrated with DNA methylation, which also differs between tissues. DNA methylation is detectable in cirDNA, making it possible to identify its origin by methylation patterns.[40,41]

PCR-based Methods for Quantifying Circulating Cell-Free DNA

Two PCR-based methods are generally used for cirDNA analyses — real-time or quantitative PCR (qPCR) and digital PCR (dPCR). Several platforms exist for both methods. In qPCR, two types of chemistry are commonly used to detect the PCR product: probe-based chemistries or dye-based chemistries. Probe-based methods utilize a fluorescently labelled probe that emits light of a certain wavelength upon cleavage during PCR amplification. Hence, an increase in fluorescence is only seen if a specific target, determined by primer sequences, is amplified and the probe matches a specific sequence between the primers. The dye-based methods rely on the specificity of the primers, and increases in fluorescence are observed when double-stranded DNA is produced during amplification and the dye intercalates the two strands. One disadvantage of the dye-based methods is that once an incorrectly primed amplification cycle has taken place, the incorrect product incorporates a perfectly matched primer sequence and forms an efficient template for further amplification rounds. Probe-based methods provide an additional level of specificity since, in addition to the primers, the probe also requires a complementary sequence to be present within the product in order for a fluorescence signal to be generated.

dPCR is now widely used for cirDNA analyses. The principle of dPCR is that samples are partitioned into a large number of reactions (10^4 to 10^7), only some of which include a template molecule. Each partition contains mastermix, primers, and probes or dye exactly as in qPCR reactions. If a template molecule is present in a partition, PCR amplification takes place and fluorescence is detected as an endpoint measurement, with individual partitions designated as positive or negative. Based on the number of positive and negative partitions, the number of template molecules in the original sample can be determined with high accuracy. The advantage of dPCR over qPCR lies mainly in the sensitivity for detecting rare targets (e.g., mutations or methylations) in a high background (e.g., wild-type or unmethylated DNA). dPCR does not require the use of standard curves or reference materials for quantification purposes, as it provides an absolute quantification of the template. It is, however, a more expensive method that is lower throughput and requires more hands-on time, so for quantification of total cirDNA, qPCR would be the preferred method for analyses of samples, with dPCR used for quantifying standards for standard curves.

For dPCR, the common approach to analyzing a point mutation is a duplex reaction with two primers and two probes, with each probe labelled with a different fluorophore. The two probes detect the wild type and mutated sequence, respectively. Because of the partitioning of the template molecules, the background is greatly reduced and assay specificity becomes less vital. The wild-type probe blocks unspecific detection of wild-type DNA by the mutation-specific probe and quantifies the number of wild-type alleles.

For analyzing point mutations or methylated sites by qPCR, specific optimizations should be employed to increase the specificity. One common approach is Amplification Refractory Mutation System qPCR (ARMS-qPCR), in which a mismatch is incorporated into one of the primer sequences next to the mutated position to improve discrimination.[42] This approach exploits the fact that while a single mismatched residue within a primer can often be tolerated, two adjacent mismatched residues render the reaction too inefficient to proceed. Wild-type blocking oligos that hybridize to the wild-type sequence and prevent DNA extension can also be added to the mutation-detecting reaction to minimize nonspecific amplification of wild-type sequences, such as the Int-plex method.[43]

Co-Amplification at Lower Denaturation Temperature PCR (COLD-PCR) is a method to enrich for templates containing a rare mutated sequence. COLD-PCR relies on a two-step dena-turation protocol. The first denaturation at 94°C is followed by DNA reannealing at around 70°C. When the mutant sequence is rare and wild-type sequence is present at a high excess, the majority of mutation-containing DNA fragments will form het-eroduplexes with the wild-type sequence. A second denaturation step is then carried out at a temperature selected to denature the heteroduplexes but not the perfectly matched homodu-plexes containing the wild-type sequence only. Single-nucleotide mismatches alter the melting temperature of double-stranded DNA slightly (0.2°C–1.5°C), and two fragments differing by only single-nucleotide mismatch will have different amplifica-tion efficiencies at the critical temperature. With this approach, amplification of the mutated sequence is favored and more eas-ily detected in a downstream application as pyrosequencing or NGS.[44] It is important to note that COLD-PCR improves the amplification of the *minor* DNA sequence, so if a sample con-tained an excess of mutant over wild-type DNA, it is the amplifi-cation of the wild-type DNA that would be enhanced.

For methylated DNA analysis, methylation is measured by bisulfite conversion of DNA followed by quantification of meth-ylated and unmethylated CpG residues by methylation-specific qPCR (e.g., the MethyLight method).[45] Developments of the method specifically for cirDNA include analyses by dPCR in order to detect smaller fractions of tumor-related DNA that exhibit a different methylation pattern.[46,47] One of the technical difficulties related to analyzing methylated cirDNA is that the bisulphite conversion process further fragments the DNA strands, leading to some loss of amplifiable template.[48]

Target Region

There are a number of considerations when selecting a target region for PCR analysis of cirDNA. If quantitation of total cancer cirDNA is required, it is important to choose a region that is known not to be amplified or deleted in the cancer of interest. It is advisable to test several different targets and compare levels.

Some genes are also present in the genome as pseudogenes and should be used with caution. PCR reactions targeting pseudogenes with multiple copies in the genome may give different results depending on whether dPCR or qPCR with a standard curve is used. This is because dPCR will directly quantitate the number of pseudogene copies, which will then need to be compared against the number of known pseudogenes in the genome in order to calculate how many genome equivalents are present in the sample. qPCR against a standard curve will directly quantitate the amount of DNA present since the genomic DNA used in the standard curve contains the same number of pseudogenes as the unknown sample. Pseudogenes only contain exons, so if one of the primers is positioned in an intron region of the gene, this should not cause problems.

When positioning primers, sequences with known polymorphisms should be avoided, in order to maintain consistent PCR efficiency in samples from different individuals. Primer dimers and hairpins should be eliminated by investigating primers in dedicated software, and a BLAST search should be performed to ensure specific primer binding. The secondary structure of the amplicon should also be checked to ensure that the primer-binding sites are without secondary structures at the annealing temperature.

When quantifying total cirDNA, there are often several options for positioning the assay along a gene or DNA region. Because the fragmentation of DNA is nonrandom, this may have implications for the quantification of cirDNA. Nucleosome distribution, and hence DNA fragmentation pattern, should be a factor in guiding positioning, if these are known or can be predicted. Assays that overlap the positions where DNA is frequently cleaved (e.g., transcription start sites) may result in lower quantifications than assays that are completely within the fragments. Gene activity, and therefore DNA fragmentation pattern, varies between tissues and the same assay could potentially perform differently in patients with different cancers. The assay could also perform differently in healthy individuals making it difficult to compare DNA quantifications to "normal" levels. DNA fragmentation may differ between patients depending on type and stage of disease. Patients with a low fraction of circulating tumor DNA have longer fragments in circulation while patients with higher fractions have shorter fragments than healthy individuals, indicating that fragmentation pattern develops with the disease.[8] This could potentially influence quantifications in patients over time and produce measured drops in the level of cirDNA that are not real. Again, it would be advisable to measure more than one target.

When analyzing tumor-specific DNA, positioning is determined by the genetic abnormality under investigation. When quantifying point mutations, the assay must cover the specific base position; when analyzing methylation, CpG residues determine the positioning. Nucleosome distribution is particularly relevant to the analysis of CpG sites in promoter-associated CpG islands.

These regions are, by their nature, adjacent to or overlapping with transcription start sites, and as such, care must be taken to avoid positioning the PCR assay over the transcription start site of active genes where nucleosomes are absent.

Analyzing copy number variations is often done by comparing quantitative values of two PCR assays from unaffected and amplified genomic regions. The two assays have to be carefully characterized and compared experimentally in order to avoid artefacts. Positioning of assays could in this case potentially influence results if the assays are not in similar positions with regard to fragmentation patterns. The same is the case with integrity analyses where two assays of different lengths are compared.

Purification

Because tumor-specific cirDNA is generally shorter than DNA derived from normal cells, it is important to use isolation and purification techniques that include short fragments. It has been shown that spike-in fragments of different lengths are not purified equally well with different purification kits[49] so the appropriate DNA capture kit needs to be selected. Kits dedicated to purification of cirDNA are often optimized for isolating short fragments to minimize contaminating genomic DNA, but longer fragments released by necrosis in some patients are also lost.

It is possible to analyze cirDNA directly from plasma without purification.[50] The amount of DNA and the integrity of the DNA change after purification and depend on the purification method. This demonstrates that it is also important to consider the purification method when comparing results from different studies. Underhill *et al.*[51] demonstrated that by size-selecting for short fragments by polyacrylamide gel electrophoresis, increases in fraction of mutated DNA could be observed. Hence, a better sensitivity for detecting genetic changes could be obtained by excluding larger fragments from the analyses.

Assay Length

According to the literature, shorter PCR assays lead to higher amounts of detectable DNA.[24,33,52] When designing assays for PCR-based analyses of cirDNA, it is evident that amplicons should be less than 166 bp long since the majority of fragments in circulation are of that size or smaller, and when optimizing analyses to be tumor specific, very short amplicons are necessary. Decreasing the size of the PCR amplicon increases the likelihood that it will fall entirely within a cirDNA fragment and not span a break point.

Quantification by qPCR is dependent on amplification efficiency, which generally increases when amplicons are shorter. This is in part because amplicon length influences how susceptible the reaction is to PCR inhibitors, with longer amplicons being more prone to inhibition.[53] When comparing quantifications by different assays, it is necessary to take this into account. In a direct comparison of quantifications with long (120 bp) and short (85 bp) assays, the short assays amplified between 2.5 and 5 times more efficiently than longer assays on the same positive control material.[54]

Because tumor-derived cirDNA is shorter than normal cirDNA, the benefit of using short assays is highest with tumor DNA.[24,33] Shortening qPCR assays specific for *KRAS*-mutated DNA from 120 to 85 bp increased the amount of DNA detected in cancer patient samples 3 times.[54] This was after taking into account that short assays performed more efficiently, so the increase is directly associated with the sample material being shorter.

The difference in amplification efficiency between assays of different lengths is of course especially important when using qPCR for calculating integrity indexes of cirDNA. Assays to analyze integrity indices are by definition of different lengths, so to determine the relative quantities of the long and short fragments, assays have to be carefully compared and variations in efficiencies taken into account. Otherwise, the result of the integrity index will depend on the total level of DNA in the sample. For example, cancer patients often have increased amounts of cirDNA, and with a longer assay being less efficient, the integrity of the DNA would appear to be increased compared to healthy controls.

If assays cannot be designed to be of identical length, standard curves can be generated to identify the amplification efficiency of each assay and quantifications can be adjusted accordingly. It would, however, be important to calculate the efficiency on standard curve material that is comparable to sample material. This means using fragmented DNA for the standard curve, but since DNA from plasma is not fragmented in a random manner, it is difficult to generate a perfectly comparable standard curve material. Ideally, DNA purified from plasma from a source with high levels of cirDNA should be used in the standard curve, but this also does not take into account individual differences in cirDNA fragmentation patterns.

Amplicons of 50–150 bp are recommended for efficient qPCR assays. For most targets, this is long enough to design primers and probes of adequate length. For probe-based qPCR methods, the minimal length of an amplicon is determined by the length of two primers and the probe. One primer and probe on one strand can be next to each other and should ideally be as close as possible without overlapping to ensure rapid cleavage by the polymerase. For dye-based assays, amplicons will often have to be slightly longer than probe-based assays in order to differentiate the PCR product from primer–dimers in the melt curve analysis. In practice, this means designing amplicons of 90–150 bp. The quantification of a template using intercalating dye depends on the length of the amplicon and the AT-content of the amplicon sequence.[55] The copy number is overestimated with long amplicons so caution should be taken when comparing different assays or comparing dye-based with probe-based methods.

Primer/Probe Design

Primers and probes have to be of a certain length to work optimally. The specificity of a primer increases with length. To avoid unspecific binding, which can significantly lower the efficiency of an assay, primers generally should be 15–25 bases. The GC content should be around 50%, and stretches of identical nucleotides should be avoided. The melting temperature (Tm) of the primers should ideally be 50°C–65°C and should not differ more than 2°C–5°C between the primers. If the Tm between primers differs more, there may not be an annealing temperature at which both primers will work optimally. The Tm is primarily affected by the primer length and GC content but also primer and salt concentration in the reaction.

The 5' position of the probe should not be a G, as this quenches the fluorescence, even after probe hydrolysis, and the GC content should be around 50%. The Tm of the probe should be 5°C–10°C higher than that of the primers. If the melting temperature of the probe is close to the Tm of the primers, the percentage of probe bound to the target will be low when primers anneal and extension begins. The primers would start to amplify a product, but since many targets would be without probe, the correct amount of target would not be measured. The Tm of a probe can be increased by using modifications such as minor groove binders (MGB), modified nucleic acids (e.g., peptide nucleic acids (PNA) or locked nucleic acids (LNA)). When designing assays for mutation detection, the mismatch should be positioned in the central third or toward the 3'end of the probe but not in the last two nucleotides.

Optimization of Short Amplicon PCR

Short amplicons are more likely to denature during the melting step of the PCR reaction, and primers and probes are more likely to bind their target. It may be possible and beneficial to shorten the length of the denaturation step after the initial cycles. Standard Taq DNA polymerase has a half-life of approximately 40 min at 95°C and hence its activity decreases slightly with every PCR cycle. Depurination events may also occur at elevated temperatures leading to mutations in the PCR product. This is, however, mainly a problem with long PCR amplicons.

It has also been demonstrated that lowering the denaturation temperature after a few initial cycles improves the yield of short PCR products when using Taq polymerase. One study showed that by lowering the temperature from 94°C to 87°C after 5–10 cycles, the yield of a 110-bp product could be increased 4–6-fold.[56] Below 90°C the half-life of Taq polymerase is significantly longer. After a few cycles, the predominant template for amplification is PCR amplicons, which denature much more readily than long genomic DNA, and consequently the denaturation temperature can be decreased. The extension step can in theory also be short, as the length of DNA to be amplified is short, and polymerases can extend DNA at a fast rate.

When quantifying cirDNA, duplicate or triplicate PCR reactions should be performed and appropriate controls should be included in each analysis. For tumor cirDNA analyses, this includes two negative controls (no template control and wild-type only DNA template) and a positive control consisting of DNA containing the tumor-specific marker diluted in wild-type DNA.

Standard curves should be generated for qPCR analyses to determine amplification efficiencies. It is difficult to generate standard curves that are completely comparable to real samples, especially for analyses for circulating tumor DNA. Samples from a patient with high levels of cirDNA may be used, but these may be extremely difficult to obtain — especially in the quantities needed to analyze standard curves a number of times and would only reflect fragmentation pattern in one patient. As an alternative, short synthetic fragments could be used. If possible, the synthetic fragments should be spiked into a plasma matrix but, if this isn't possible, they can be spiked into fragmented genomic DNA.

Primer quality and batch variation should be monitored over time by plotting Cq values or quantitative measurements for control samples. It is important to use high-quality primers and probes and store them correctly, as this can dramatically influence amplification efficiency and lead to very different Cq values. In dPCR, variation in primer/probe batches is less of a challenge because the quantification is performed as an end-point measurement. Fluorescence levels could be different for different batches of primers and probes, but the overall quantification would generally be identical.

Other optimizations can be investigated to improve discrimination between tumor and wild-type DNA. Lower dNTP levels, higher annealing temperatures, lower primer, $MgCl_2$, and enzyme concentrations all increase the stringency of the amplification and favor amplification of the sequence that correctly matches the primers.

Conclusions

Many factors influence analyses of cirDNA by PCR-based methods. The fragmented nature of the DNA is particularly important to take into account when designing and validating assays. The positioning and length of amplicon can greatly influence the analysis and care must be taken when comparing results from different assays.

The current knowledge about biological properties of cirDNA is difficult to implement in designing PCR assays for cirDNA analyses, but in future, more applicable knowledge about fragmentation patterns and release mechanisms with regard to disease type and severity may become available.

Many resources are put into finding clinical applications for cirDNA analyses. Research into the origin and biology of cirDNA is equally important and necessary in order to develop the most relevant and clinically useful analyses with regard to specific patient groups.

References

1. Lui YY, Chik KW, Chiu RW, Ho CY, *et al.* (2002) Predominant hematopoietic origin of cell-free DNA in plasma and serum after sex-mismatched bone marrow transplantation. *Clin Chem* **48**: 421–427.
2. Peters DL, Pretorius PJ. (2011) Origin, translocation and destination of extracellular occurring DNA — a new paradigm in genetic behaviour. *Clin Chim Acta* **412**: 806–811.
3. Thierry AR, El Messaoudi S, Gahan PB, *et al.* (2016) Origins, structures, and functions of circulating DNA in oncology. *Cancer Metastasis Rev* **35**: 347–376.

4. Beck J, Urnovitz HB, Riggert J, *et al.* (2009) Profile of the circulating DNA in apparently healthy individuals. *Clin Chem* **55**: 730–738.

5. Morozkin ES, Loseva EM, Morozov IV, *et al.* (2012) A comparative study of cell-free apoptotic and genomic DNA using FISH and massive parallel sequencing. *Expert Opin Biol Ther* **12**: S11–S17.

6. Stroun M, Lyautey J, Lederrey C, *et al.* (2001) Alu repeat sequences are present in increased proportions compared to a unique gene in plasma/serum DNA: Evidence for a preferential release from viable cells? *Ann N Y Acad Sci* **945**: 258–264.

7. Jahr S, Hentze H, Englisch S, *et al.* (2001) DNA fragments in the blood plasma of cancer patients: Quantitations and evidence for their origin from apoptotic and necrotic cells. *Cancer Res* **61**: 1659–1665.

8. Jiang P, Chan CW, Chan KC, *et al.* (2015) Lengthening and shortening of plasma DNA in hepatocellular carcinoma patients. *Proc Natl Acad Sci U S A* **112**: E1317–E1325.

9. Zheng YW, Chan KC, Sun H, *et al.* (2012) Nonhematopoietically derived DNA is shorter than hematopoietically derived DNA in plasma: A transplantation model. *Clin Chem* **58**: 549–558.

10. Burnham P, Kim MS, Agbor-Enoh S, *et al.* (2016) Single-stranded DNA library preparation uncovers the origin and diversity of ultrashort cell-free DNA in plasma. *Sci Rep* **6**: 27859.

11. Mouliere F, El MS, Pang D, *et al.* (2014) Multi-marker analysis of circulating cell-free DNA toward personalized medicine for colorectal cancer. *Mol Oncol* **8**: 927–941.

12. Snyder MW, Kircher M, Hill AJ, *et al.* (2016) Cell-free DNA comprises an *in vivo* nucleosome footprint that informs its tissues-of-origin. *Cell* **164**: 57–68.

13. Schones DE, Cui K, Cuddapah S, *et al.* (2008) Dynamic regulation of nucleosome positioning in the human genome. *Cell* **132**: 887–898.

14. Struhl K, Segal E. (2013) Determinants of nucleosome positioning. *Nat Struct Mol Biol* **20**: 267–273.

15. Ma X, Zhu L, Wu X, *et al.* (2017) Cell-free DNA provides a good representation of the tumor genome despite its biased fragmentation patterns. *PLoS One* **12**: e0169231.

16. Andersson R, Enroth S, Rada-Iglesias A, *et al.* (2009) Nucleosomes are well positioned in exons and carry characteristic histone modifications. *Genome Res* **19**: 1732–1741.

17. Chodavarapu RK, Feng S, Bernatavichute YV, *et al.* (2010) Relationship between nucleosome positioning and DNA methylation. *Nature* **466**: 388–392.

18. Schwartz S, Meshorer E, Ast G. (2009) Chromatin organization marks exon-intron structure. *Nat Struct Mol Biol* **16**: 990–995.

19. Lander ES, Linton LM, Birren B, *et al.* (2001) Initial sequencing and analysis of the human genome. *Nature* **409**: 860–921.

20. Chandrananda D, Thorne NP, Bahlo M. (2015) High-resolution characterization of sequence signatures due to non-random cleavage of cell-free DNA. *BMC Med Genomics* **8**: 29.

21. Ivanov M, Baranova A, Butler T, *et al.* (2015) Non-random fragmentation patterns in circulating cell-free DNA reflect epigenetic regulation. *BMC Genomics* **16**: S1.

22. Zhang R, Nakahira K, Guo X, *et al.* (2016) Very short mitochondrial DNA fragments and heteroplasmy in human plasma. *Sci Rep* **6**: 36097.

23. Warton K, Mahon KL, Samimi G. (2016) Methylated circulating tumor DNA in blood: Power in cancer prognosis and response. *Endocr Relat Cancer* **23**: R157–R171.

24. Diehl F, Li M, Dressman D, *et al.* (2005) Detection and quantification of mutations in the plasma of patients with colorectal tumors. *Proc Natl Acad Sci USA* **102**: 16368–16373.

25. Spindler KL, Appelt AL, Pallisgaard N, *et al.* (2014) Cell-free DNA in healthy individuals, non-cancerous disease and strong prognostic value in colorectal cancer. *Int J Cancer* **135**: 2984–2991.

26. Fleischhacker M, Schmidt B. (2007) Circulating Nucleic Acids (CNAs) and cancer — a survey. *Biochim Biophys Acta* **1775**: 181–232.

27. Bettegowda C, Sausen M, Leary RJ, *et al.* (2014) Detection of circulating tumor DNA in early- and late-stage human malignancies. *Sci Transl Med* **6**: 224ra24.

28. Siravegna G, Bardelli A. (2014) Genotyping cell-free tumor DNA in the blood to detect residual disease and drug resistance. *Genome Biol* **15**: 449.

29. Hanley R, Rieger-Christ KM, Canes D, *et al.* (2006) DNA integrity assay: A plasma-based screening tool for the detection of prostate cancer. *Clin Cancer Res* **12**: 4569–4574.

30. Jiang WW, Zahurak M, Goldenberg D, *et al.* (2006) Increased plasma DNA integrity index in head and neck cancer patients. *Int J Cancer* **119**: 2673–2676.

31. Umetani N, Kim J, Hiramatsu S, *et al.* (2006) Increased integrity of free circulating DNA in sera of patients with colorectal or periampullary cancer: Direct quantitative PCR for ALU repeats. *Clin Chem* **52**: 1062–1069.

32. Wang BG, Huang HY, Chen YC, *et al.* (2003) Increased plasma DNA integrity in cancer patients. *Cancer Res* **63**: 3966–3968.

33. Mouliere F, Robert B, Arnau PE, *et al.* (2011) High fragmentation characterizes tumour-derived circulating DNA. *PLoSOne* **6**: e23418.

34. Diaz LA, Jr., Bardelli A. (2014) Liquid biopsies: Genotyping circulating tumor DNA. *J Clin Oncol* **32**: 579–586.

35. Madhavan D, Wallwiener M, Bents K, *et al.* (2014) Plasma DNA integrity as a biomarker for primary and metastatic breast cancer and potential marker for early diagnosis. *Breast Cancer Res Treat* **146**: 163–174.

36. Umetani N, Giuliano AE, Hiramatsu SH, *et al.* (2006) Prediction of breast tumor progression by integrity of free circulating DNA in serum. *J Clin Oncol* **24**: 4270–4276.

37. Ellinger J, Muller SC, Wernert N, *et al.* (2008) Mitochondrial DNA in serum of patients with prostate cancer: A predictor of biochemical recurrence after prostatectomy. *BJU Int* **102**: 628–632.

38. Mahmoud EH, Fawzy A, Ahmad OK, Ali AM. (2015) Plasma circulating cell-free nuclear and mitochondrial DNA as potential biomarkers in the peripheral blood of breast cancer patients. *Asian Pac J Cancer Prev* **16**: 8299–8305.

39. Mehra N, Penning M, Maas J, *et al.* (2007) Circulating mitochondrial nucleic acids have prognostic value for survival in patients with advanced prostate cancer. *Clin Cancer Res* **13**: 421–426.

40. Lehmann-Werman R, Neiman D, Zemmour H, *et al.* (2016) Identification of tissue-specific cell death using methylation patterns of circulating DNA. *Proc Natl Acad Sci U S A* **113**: E1826–E1834.

41. Sun K, Jiang P, Chan KC, *et al.* (2015) Plasma DNA tissue mapping by genome-wide methylation sequencing for noninvasive prenatal, cancer, and transplantation assessments. *Proc Natl Acad Sci U S A* **112**: E5503–E5512.

42. Newton CR, Graham A, Heptinstall LE, *et al.* (1989) Analysis of any point mutation in DNA. The Amplification Refractory Mutation System (ARMS). *Nucleic Acids Res* **17**: 2503–2516.

43. Mouliere F, El Messaoudi S, Gongora C, *et al.* (2013) Circulating cell-free DNA from colorectal cancer patients may reveal high KRAS or BRAF mutation load. *Transl Oncol* **6**: 319–328.

44. Tost J. (2016) The clinical potential of enhanced-ice-COLD-PCR. *Expert Rev Mol Diagn* **16**: 265–268.

45. Eads CA, Danenberg KD, Kawakami K, *et al.* (2000) MethyLight: A high-throughput assay to measure DNA methylation. *Nucleic Acids Res* **28**: E32.

46. Garrigou S, Perkins G, Garlan F, *et al.* (2016) A study of hypermethylated circulating tumor DNA as a universal colorectal cancer biomarker. *Clin Chem* **62**: 1129–1139.

47. Li M, Chen WD, Papadopoulos N, *et al.* (2009) Sensitive digital quantification of DNA methylation in clinical samples. *Nat Biotechnol* **27**: 858–863.

48. Worm Orntoft MB, Jensen SO, Hansen TB, *et al.* (2017) Comparative analysis of 12 different kits for bisulfite conversion of circulating cell-free DNA. *Epigenetics* **12**: 626–636.

49. Devonshire AS, Whale AS, Gutteridge A, *et al.* (2014) Towards standardisation of cell-free DNA measurement in plasma: Controls for extraction efficiency, fragment size bias and quantification. *Anal Bioanal Chem* **406**: 6499–6512.

50. Breitbach S, Tug S, Helmig S, *et al.* (2014) Direct quantification of cell-free, circulating DNA from unpurified plasma. *PLoS One* **9**: e87838.

51. Underhill HR, Kitzman JO, Hellwig S, *et al.* (2016) Fragment length of circulating tumor DNA. *PLoS Genet* **12**: e1006162.

52. Suzawa K, Yamamoto H, Ohashi K, *et al.* (2017) Optimal method for quantitative detection of plasma EGFR T790M mutation using droplet digital PCR system. *Oncol Rep* **37**: 3100–3106.

53. Pionzio AM, McCord BR. (2014) The effect of internal control sequence and length on the response to PCR inhibition in real-time PCR quantitation. *Forensic Sci Int Genet* **9**: 55–60.

54. Andersen RF, Spindler KL, Brandslund I, *et al.* (2015) Improved sensitivity of circulating tumor DNA measurement using short PCR amplicons. *Clin Chim Acta* **439**: 97–101.

55. Colborn JM, Byrd BD, Koita OA, Krogstad DJ. (2008) Estimation of copy number using SYBR Green: Confounding by AT-rich DNA and by variation in amplicon length. *Am J Trop Med Hyg* **79**: 887–892.

56. Yap EP, McGee JO. (1991) Short PCR product yields improved by lower denaturation temperatures. *Nucleic Acids Res* **19**: 1713.

Chapter 6

Preparation of Next-Generation Sequencing Libraries for Sequencing Circulating DNA

Katrin Heider, Florent Mouliere and Christopher G. Smith

Abstract

Next-generation sequencing of circulating DNA brings a set of challenges distinct to sequencing genomic DNA, stemming largely from its low-concentration and heavily fragmented nature. This chapter considers different approaches to sequencing library preparation, and how these are tailored to circulating DNA analysis.

Challenges Associated with Circulating Tumor DNA Analysis

Circulating cell-free DNA (cirDNA) that is found in the circulation has emerged as a biomarker of choice to monitor and track cancer in a minimally invasive manner. The portion of cirDNA that originates from tumor cells is termed circulating tumor DNA (ctDNA).[1,2] ctDNA can capture the global representation of the cancer that might be missed using a standard biopsy procedure.[3-5]

The minimally invasive nature of the approach also allows for longitudinal sampling, which is less harmful than using CT scans or biopsies.[1,2,6,7]

Due to the nature, structure, and concentration of cirDNA in the blood, sequencing of cirDNA requires optimized preparation methods. Sensitivity for ctDNA detection is hampered by the low amounts of DNA released in the bloodstream by tumor cells, as well as by the technological and conceptual limitations.[2] The main challenge in ctDNA detection is to distinguish mutant ctDNA released by the tumor from the generally overwhelming quantities of cirDNA that originates from healthy cells in the body. This distinction becomes easier with a higher concentration of ctDNA, which is related to cancer type and stage of disease.[8-10] Bettegowda and colleagues showed that the detectability of ctDNA with a PCR-based assay or Safe-SeqS, a massively parallel sequencing method, was close to 100% in the plasma of advanced bladder, colorectal, gastroesophageal, and ovarian cancer patients.[9] In these cases, the concentration of ctDNA was high enough to allow for detection of mutant fragments. On the other hand, for advanced glioma or for kidney cancer patients, the average rate of detection was only around 10%, and the concentration of ctDNA detected was also minimal (less than 10 copies per 5 mL of plasma in glioblastoma patients).[9] The lower levels of ctDNA in these cancers have since been confirmed in other studies.[11,12]

ctDNA is thought to be released via apoptosis, necrosis, proliferation, or active secretion.[2,5,13] With an increase in tumor volume, common for later stage disease, there is a concomitant increase in the number of cancerous cells with the potential to release ctDNA. It could also be hypothesized that the surface of contact of these cells with blood vessels will be increased, favoring the release of DNA fragments in the blood. For high-grade serous ovarian carcinoma, it was demonstrated that the overall volume of the tumor is strongly correlated with the levels of ctDNA measured in plasma.[14] A similar trend was later confirmed for lung cancer patients at earlier disease stages with lower tumor burden.[5] Analysis of ctDNA samples from certain cancer types or at earlier stage of disease may require more sensitive methods of analysis.

Another challenge in the analysis of ctDNA is that it is highly fragmented in plasma and other body fluids. The length of plasma cirDNA fragments is organized around a mode of 166 bp, representing the length of DNA wrapped around the nucleosome and a linker histone.[15] This mode of distribution is usually complemented by additional peaks at multiples of 166 bp, representing di- and trinucleosomes, typical of an apoptotic ladder.[16,17] As compared to cirDNA, ctDNA has been shown to be even more fragmented, exhibiting a mode of distribution between 133 and 145 bp (or smaller) in length.[11,18,19] Due to the cleavage of DNA by nucleases during cell death, the composition of bases at the ends of cirDNA fragments is also altered in cancer compared to healthy controls.[20]

There are multiple sequencing-based methods that can be used to analyze cirDNA. The techniques differ in the way the library is prepared, the size of the genome that will be analyzed, and the mean sequencing depth per sample. In the following sections, we will compare different methods for cirDNA library preparation and sequencing, highlighting the advantages and disadvantages associated with each.

Preparing Next-Generation Sequencing Libraries from Cell-Free DNA

Multiple strategies are currently available to prepare a DNA sample for next-generation sequencing. Both digital polymerase chain reaction (dPCR) and library preparation methods are commonly used in ctDNA analysis; however, this chapter will mostly focus on the latter. Library preparation usually entails sample fragmentation of genomic DNA followed by end repair, appending sequencer-specific "adapters" to fragments, and amplification.[21] Due to the fragmented nature of cirDNA and the generally low levels of ctDNA, library preparation protocols differ from those used in analysis of genomic DNA. For this chapter, we will focus on preparation of libraries for sequencing on Illumina platforms. However, there are alternative sequencers currently, or soon to become, available with their own sample preparation requirements/protocols.[22]

Quantification of Cell-Free DNA Prior to Library Preparation

Before initiating cirDNA library preparation, it is important to accurately determine the number of cirDNA molecules present in a sample. The most commonly used methods in the ctDNA field involve quantification through the use of fluorescent dyes (using equipment like Thermo Fisher's Qubit), PCR (quantitative PCR — qPCR or digital PCR — dPCR), or microfluidic DNA gel electrophoresis (using equipment like Agilent's Bioanalyzer).[23] The main differences in these methods are with respect to cost, ease and time of handling, and reproducibility. PCR approaches are more reproducible than fluorescent dye approaches but come at a higher cost and more complex setup.[24] Especially for samples at lower cirDNA concentration qPCR is the more appropriate method since it is more robust and reproducible.[23,24]

While fluorescent dye or gel separation techniques quantify the total amounts of genomic material, dPCR quantifies the number of DNA copies in a given sample by quantifying a specific region in a gene (usually a housekeeping gene is chosen).[25] As cancer is a disease that often results in changes in copy number, this may present a problem for dPCR-based quantification, as the total levels of cirDNA will not necessarily correspond to the number of genome equivalents present in the plasma. As such, it may be more appropriate to average the inferred concentration as determined by dPCR of multiple genomic loci.[26,27] Despite this concern, dPCR generally represents a more accurate measure of the concentration of a given sample. Therefore, it is advisable to quantify the sample using dPCR, even if the fragmented nature of cirDNA prevents a direct conversion of the detected number of copies by dPCR into nanograms of DNA.

Library Preparation from DNA

In general, library preparation involves end repair to create molecules with blunt ends, which is followed by adapter ligation and PCR amplification.[28,29] This final step is generally necessary due to the low concentrations of input DNA that are commonly available from cirDNA.[28,30] One of the main challenges when sequencing DNA libraries is to mitigate the bias introduced by PCR amplification.[29] This challenge is particularly important in cancer genomics when attempting to sensitively detect single-nucleotide variants (SNVs) targetable by precision medicine.[31] Another consideration is the maintenance of molecular complexity during library preparation to increase the chances of finding rare mutations with low allelic frequencies. Current methods typically vary in the efficiency with which the final output represents the molecules that went into the reaction.[29,30]

Double-Stranded DNA Library Preparation

The most commonly used library preparation protocols in the cirDNA field are aimed at sequencing double-stranded DNA. Indeed, a multitude of kits and methods are available that follow a similar workflow. While tissue or germline DNA library preparation kits require a fragmentation step to generate short fragments (~200 bp) compatible with the sequencer (a potential source of severe fragment loss),[32] cirDNA samples do not have to undergo DNA shearing due to its already fragmented nature. The cirDNA sample first undergoes end repair, followed by phosphorylation of the 5' prime ends. The 3' ends undergo an A-tailing step to allow for ligation of the sequencer-specific adapters. Upon adapter ligation, samples undergo several cycles of PCR to enrich the fragments that are compatible with the sequencer. This is followed by a final "cleanup" of the library to remove excess adapter dimers and heteroduplexes.[29,32,33] Individual DNA samples can be tagged with uniquely barcoded adapters. These barcodes consist of a short and unique stretch of bases and allow for multiplexed sequencing. Molecules originating from the same sample will obtain the same string of unique bases; therefore, each barcoded DNA fragment in the sequencing pool can be attributed to its sample of origin.[31]

Competition in the market of library preparation kits has helped to lower the prices while also improving their quality. The required input for most kits starts at less than a nanogram of DNA, allowing for sample preparation even when very little material is available.[30]

The most commonly used double-stranded library preparation protocols tend to capture fragments greater than 100 bp in length.[34] It is still unclear why shorter fragments are not observed but there are different hypotheses. Shorter molecules could be lost during the extraction or library clean up steps, or be damaged or of single-stranded nature and thereby not captured by the double-stranded protocol. This results in the loss of fragments shorter than 100 bp, which may be enriched for ctDNA.[18,19] Single-stranded library preparation methods have emerged as an alternative library preparation approach that may overcome this problem.[34,35]

Single-Stranded DNA Library Preparation

Developed for the analysis of ancient, degraded DNA, current single-stranded DNA library preparation methods allow for the capture of single-stranded, double-stranded, and damaged DNA fragments.[35] Therefore, as compared to double-stranded library preparation protocols that capture only double-stranded DNA, single-stranded DNA library preparation allows for the analysis of a broader range of DNA fragments. Indeed, in a study that used a single-stranded protocol on DNA from a cohort of transplant patients, a greater portion of 50–100 bp fragments was recovered using this approach as compared to a double-stranded equivalent.[34] Also, when applied to plasma samples from healthy individuals, a greater representation of shorter DNA fragments was recovered as compared to the standard double-stranded library preparation.[36] An updated version of the Gansauge and Meyer ancient DNA protocol was published in 2017, showing greater recovery of DNA and an improved turn-around time.[37] Previous research suggested an enrichment of ctDNA in shorter fragments.[18,19,38,39] Therefore, the use of single-stranded DNA library preparation protocols that improve the coverage of shorter fragments might be expected to improve the recovery, and detection, of ctDNA. However, initial reports seem to indicate that there is no improvement in ctDNA detection using a single-stranded DNA library,[40] raising questions as to the origin of the additional DNA fragments that are captured by this protocol.

Other single-stranded protocols include the commercially available SMART ChIP-Seq kit that is based on template switching. This protocol was initially developed for RNA approaches.[41,42] Compared to the ancient DNA protocols described previously, the SMART ChIP–Seq protocol involves a simpler, and quicker, workflow. However, a recent publication indicates that this method preferentially captures fragments with poly dA/dT tracts, which could induce a bias in cirDNA recovery.[43] Similar comparisons should be performed on the other library preparation methods to obtain a clearer picture of the sequencing biases specific to each method.

Enrichment of ctDNA

While single-stranded library preparation protocols aid in capturing shorter DNA fragments, which might be biased toward a higher proportion of ctDNA, they do not actually enrich for ctDNA. One means by which one could potentially do so is by carrying out size selection, either through in vitro or in silico means. This is based on the observation that ctDNA fragments are predominantly shorter than 150 bp, while cirDNA of noncancerous origin is predominantly 166 bp in length.[11,15,18,19,39,44,45] Such approaches have indeed shown an improvement in ctDNA detection.[11,19,40,45] In addition to size selection, methods leveraging the thermodynamic properties of primers for sequencing also enable enrichment in tumor signal.[46]

While selecting for certain fragments may lead to more confident mutation detection, the general level of background noise remains a challenge. Indeed, with an error rate of just below 1%, current sequencing yields data with high background noise.[32,47] Additionally, given the low concentration of cirDNA, PCR amplification is usually warranted during library preparation. This further leads to the introduction of PCR errors that may reach allelic fractions as high or higher than true mutations.[48,49] Methods have evolved to aid in the downstream analysis and differentiation of true mutations from noise.

Sequencing Error Correction Using Unique Molecular Identifiers

The concept of uniquely tagging individual molecules was first described in 2003 in the context of determining the unique number of mRNA molecules in a given sample.[50] In 2011, unique molecular identifiers (UMIs) were first used to reduce PCR background noise and obtain a cleaner sequencing result.[51,52] UMIs are composed of a string of entirely random nucleotides that tag each molecule of the initial sample in a unique way.[51] After sequencing, the UMIs are used to group fragments of the same origin into families, which are then combined into a single consensus sequence.[53] As shown in Fig. 1, this consensus sequence aids in identifying PCR and sequencing errors, which should only be present in some, but not all, members of a given family. Conversely, true mutations should be represented in most, if not all, of the members of that family. Thus, the use of UMIs allows for error suppression and more stringent and confident calling, which improves downstream analyses.

UMIs have made an impact within the field of ctDNA research. Examples of their application include the Safe–SeqS approach with an error rate of only 3.5×10^{-6} mutations/bp (70-fold

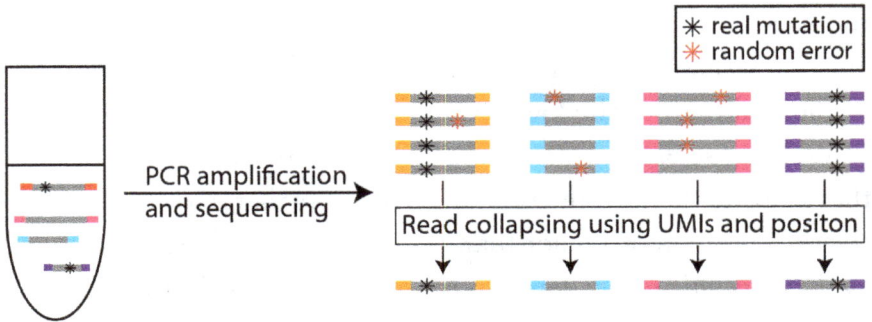

Fig. 1: Schematic representation of background noise reduction through UMIs. Unique molecules are tagged with different adapters before undergoing PCR amplification and sequencing. Utilizing read position and UMI sequence information, PCR and sequencing errors are removed and molecules are collapsed into a consensus sequence.

less than without using UMIs), which was used for a multicancer study led by Bettegowda and colleagues.[9,48] UMIs were also incorporated into the iDES CAPP–Seq approach used by Newman and colleagues to study early-stage lung cancers. Using this approach, the authors showed that, together with in-silico background "polishing," a sensitivity of 0.0025% could be achieved.[54]

Despite their promise, there are some limitations when using UMIs. For example, it is possible that PCR errors that occur early in the amplification process may not be filtered out. Furthermore, sequencing errors in the sequence of the UMI itself may lead to assignment of fragments to the wrong family.[47]

The widespread development of high-depth sequencing for ctDNA mutation analysis, as well as the availability of standardized kits, leads to an easier implementation of the approach without the necessity of prior experience.[55] Tools such as CONNOR, MAGERI, UMI-tools, and Agilent's SureCall further aid with the analysis of UMI data.[53,56–58]

Building upon the background noise suppression achieved through the use of UMIs, Schmitt and colleagues developed a technique called duplex sequencing. They not only incorporate UMIs into their library preparation but also retain strand directionality and origin to further reduce background noise.[59] After generating a strand-based consensus sequence, they identify which two strands came from the same original double-stranded molecule and combine those two consensus strands into a final duplex consensus sequence. They estimate their error rate to be at 3.8 × 10^{-10} or even lower, allowing for very sensitive mutation calling. However, this degree of read combining warrants a great initial sequencing depth, resulting in a much increased sequencing cost.[59] More recently, Cohen and colleagues developed an approach (SaferSeqS,[60] a spin-off of the SafeSeq approach described earlier) that applies identical barcodes to both strands of the input DNA fragment before strand-specific hemi-nested PCR enrichment. Mutations can be assigned to the Watson and Crick strands — those called in both strands are considered bonafide mutations. As with the approach developed by Schmitt and colleagues,[59] SaferSeqS achieves impressive sensitivity and specificity, detecting variants at frequencies below 1 in 100,000.

PCR-Free Library Preparation

In 2015, Karlsson and colleagues described a library preparation method for cirDNA and noninvasive prenatal diagnosis that does not require a PCR step.[61] Their method not only avoids amplification bias induced through PCR but also removes any errors that PCR would have produced. Based on the single-stranded library preparation introduced by Gansauge and colleagues, the authors altered the protocol to remove any PCR amplification steps.[35,61] Unlike other kits that employ PCR-free library preparation and that require more than 500 ng input material, the method proposed by Karlsson and colleagues requires only 50 ng input making it a feasible method for the analysis of cirDNA,[61] although the amount is still fairly large in the context of typical cirDNA yields. Comparing their method to a normal double-stranded library preparation protocol, as well as a UMI approach, the authors concluded that the amplification-free library preparation process increases coverage and decreases GC bias. Finally, it also retains strand information, which is otherwise lost during PCR-based library preparation.[61] The authors highlight that their method is most suitable for degraded samples and samples requiring suffi-cient coverage. When accurate sequencing is needed, for example, rare mutation detection in samples with low levels of ctDNA, they would still recommend a UMI-based approach.[61]

Other library preparation methods also aid in reducing PCR and sequencing errors but have limited applications in the field of cirDNA so far. Examples are multiple displacement amplification (MDA) and rolling circle amplification (RCA).[47,62]

Having highlighted the main options and new developments available for cirDNA library preparation, ctDNA enrichment, and error rate reduction, we will now turn toward the different sequencing methods available for cirDNA analysis.

Tailoring Approaches for Cell-Free DNA Sequencing

Upon generation of a library, different sequencing methods are available depending on the required analysis. One can either pro-ceed directly with whole genome sequencing (WGS) or enrich the sample for some part of the genome. In the following sections, different sequencing approaches will be explained in more detail and their advantages and disadvantages, as well as their applica-tion to the study of plasma DNA, will be discussed. We will group the different methods based on the size of the genome they target and provide an overview of the main differences between them.

Whole Genome Sequencing

WGS of plasma DNA provides researchers with a comprehensive view of the entire genome of the patient,[63] facilitating the analysis of somatic copy number variations (CNVs), structural variants (SVs), and SNVs. With the development of digital karyotyping, it has become possible to analyze copy number changes of the genome in greater detail, even with sufficient sensitivity to observe focal events involving small genomic regions (<1M bp).[64] Digital karyotyping laid the foundation for later copy number analysis and its implementation to plasma analysis. WGS of cancerous plasma samples was first employed in 2012 when CNVs were identified, even in the absence of matched tumor specimens.[65] Using CNVs to detect cancer represents a very useful tool since amplifications and deletions are often an early event in cancer development.[66] Additionally, it is possible to infer copy number status from low-depth data, even with a sequencing depth of $<1x$, in turn allowing simple and cost-effective interrogation of ctDNA.[67,68] The ability to detect CNVs at low depth has led to the use of terms such as shallow whole genome sequencing (sWGS) or low-pass WGS.

For sWGS-based CNV analysis, the genome is apportioned into "bins" of an equally sized length (ranging from kb to Mb). The sequencing reads that map within each of these bins are counted and this value is compared to the average bin read count across the entire genome. Any bins spanning regions that are amplified or deleted will contain greater or fewer reads than the respective average bin count. Such a ratio is obtained for every bin across the length of the genome, generating a CNV profile. This graphic representation of the genome allows one to quickly visualize amplifications and deletions, as well as compares the overall pattern between different samples from the same patient, or between different patients. The chosen bin size is dependent on the sequencing depth, where greater sequencing depth allows for a smaller bin size and, therefore, a more detailed CNV profile.

One can convert the above CNV profiles into quantifiable metrics, for example, using a z-score as described by Heitzer and colleagues.[69] This method determines a score for each sample based on the deviation in read distribution from a cohort of control plasma samples.[69] A sequencing depth coverage of 0.1× to 0.2× is sufficient to determine the z-score of a patient.[69] Other tools regularly used for quantifying ctDNA, based on CNV profiles, include tMAD[11] and ichorCNA.[67] In addition to CNV, the cirDNA fragmentation patterns could also be converted as a quantitative metric to assess tumor fraction.[70]

One can also call SNVs from WGS data; however, greater sequencing depth is needed to ensure sufficient confidence in mutation calling. Indeed, the detection limit of SNVs is directly correlated with the coverage; the more a sample is sequenced, the lower the mutation frequency detection threshold (i.e., greater sensitivity). At a sequencing depth of 17×, Chan and colleagues were able to identify both CNVs and SNVs in plasma samples from four patients with hepatocellular carcinoma and one patient with both ovarian and breast cancers.[3] Comparing the copy number data from plasma and matched tumor tissue, the authors observed a better correlation with increasing tumor size and ctDNA fraction in the plasma.[3] For the patient with breast and ovarian cancers, CNV analysis suggested that the copy number alterations of both the breast and ovarian lesions could be detected in plasma, demonstrating that plasma analysis has the potential to overcome spatial tumor heterogeneity.[3]

Furthermore, the concordance between SNV calls of the plasma and tumor samples of the hepatocellular carcinoma patients was between 15% and 94%, respectively, and was probably related to tumor size and ctDNA concentration in the plasma.[3] For the patient with ovarian and breast cancers, the authors showed that mutations shared between different tumor regions were better represented in the plasma, as reflected by their higher allele fraction.[3] Conversely, sub-clonal tumor mutations were less well-represented and had a greater chance of being missed.[3,67]

While depth of sequencing can prohibit SNV calling due to low depth, Landau and colleagues developed an approach (MRDetect)[71] that relies on integration of patient-specific somatic SNVs (as identified by prior sequencing of matched tumour tissue) across the entire breadth of sequencing for sensitive detection of ctDNA to fractions as low as parts per 10^{-5}. The sensitivity of MRDetect is related to the overall mutation rate in the sample of interest and will be better for cancers with high mutation rates such as melanoma and lung.

As outlined previously, WGS is a powerful tool to obtain genome-wide information for a sample. However, use of this tool becomes increasingly cost prohibitive as the required depth of sequencing increases. Indeed, even a modest overall depth of ~30× (generally used to genotype polymorphisms) typically has a high enough sequencing cost such as to preclude use in most clinical and research settings.

Capture-Based Sequencing Approaches

While WGS of plasma DNA can provide a comprehensive overview of a patient's genome, it lacks sensitivity for the detection of low-frequency mutations. By restricting the size of the region to be analyzed, one can reach a greater depth per sample while maintaining or decreasing the cost of sequencing. This greater depth results in a greater sensitivity and the ability to reliably detect mutations at lower frequencies.[63] After library preparation, samples can undergo a "hybrid capture" process. In this method, regions of interest are selected by the annealing of complementary DNA or RNA "baits" or primer pairs. Captured regions are amplified while uncaptured regions are washed away. Depending on the design of the capture baits, the captured regions may include the entire exome (whole exome sequencing, WES), or some other custom-designed region (custom capture sequencing). In the case of the latter, current approaches typically target commonly mutated genes, or already identified mutations.

A major limitation of capture-based approaches can be uneven coverage, due to the fact that some regions lack complexity and are difficult to target. As a result, they will not be captured and enriched as well during the hybridization, making their analysis more difficult.[72] WGS does not include a capture step, resulting in a more even and less biased coverage of the genome.

Whole Exome Sequencing

Assuming that most driver mutations will occur in the actively transcribed part of the genome, targeting the exome allows researchers to focus their sequencing efforts on this ~1% of the genome. Many companies offer exome capture reagents, varying in the capture approach, complexity of the protocol, and covered regions.[73]

WES has been demonstrated to be a useful tool for monitoring tumor evolution. Murtaza and colleagues applied WES to serial plasma samples with high (>10%) levels of ctDNA. An input of 2.3 ng DNA (690 haploid genome equivalents) and a sequencing depth of 31–160× was sufficient to call mutations from patient plasma.[4] Using longitudinally obtained samples, it was possible to track tumor evolution throughout treatment.[4]

Furthermore, Girotti and colleagues applied WES to plasma samples from stage III melanoma patients. They were able to successfully identify resistance mutations, highlighting the potential for ctDNA as a disease monitoring tool.[74] Dietz and colleagues showed the utility of WES on low-volume serum samples from stage III nonsmall cell lung cancer patients (NSCLC). However, due to limited sample input and sequencing depth (68×) they validated only 17% of mutations identified in matched tumor specimens.[75] Nevertheless, they also identified a potential resistance mutation that was absent in the corresponding tumor sample, which could explain why treatment for that patient became ineffective.[75] WES was applied to plasma samples from metastatic cancer patients in a study by Butler and colleagues.[76] They showed good correlation between tumor and plasma mutations and again identified additional plasma mutations that were absent in the tumor sample.[76] However, their study focused on only two patients, utilizing 15 mL and 25 mL of plasma at sequencing depths of 309× and 561×, respectively.[76]

While there are a growing number of studies showing the feasibility of WES on plasma and serum samples, it is important to consider the current limitations. All studies thus far have focused on later-stage cancer patients, in whom levels of ctDNA are generally higher.[9,10] Additionally, the sequencing depth in these studies is quite high which, while allowing for greater sensitivity in mutation calling, increases the overall cost of this approach. Applied to a larger cohort or in a clinical setting, WES would generally not be currently feasible.

Custom Capture Sequencing

As an alternative to "off the shelf" exome capture kits, custom capture methods have emerged, allowing one to focus sequencing efforts on particular genomic loci of interest. This, in turn, means that either the same number of samples can be sequenced to a greater depth, allowing for more sensitive mutation calling, or more samples can be sequenced to the same depth, enabling application to larger cohorts.

Cancer Personalized Profiling by Deep Sequencing (CAPP–Seq) is one example of a custom capture sequencing approach that relies on the presence of recurring mutations across a cancer cohort. Using publicly available WES, exon, and structural rearrangement data, common mutations and rearrangements are identified and used to design a targeted gene panel.[77] Focusing on NSCLC, a 125-kb panel was designed and applied to plasma samples from stage I–IV patients. The small panel size allowed for deep sequencing (~10,000× in this study) at a reasonable cost per sample. For later-stage patients, CAPP–Seq showed 100% sensitivity for ctDNA detection and proved advantageous over imaging technology for disease detection, emphasizing the potential of capture-based methods for cancer diagnosis and monitoring.[77] The same authors further developed the iDES CAPP–Seq described previously, a technique that implements molecular barcodes and polishing of sequencing "noise." These developments allow for a sensitivity of 0.0025%, sufficient for the detection of ctDNA at very low levels.[9,54]

The recent TRACERx study used patient-specific amplicon sequencing panels for the enrichment of libraries to improve detection and sensitivity.[5] Based on WES tumor data, a median of 18 SNVs were identified for each of 96 patients. These regions were enriched in libraries prepared from plasma samples. While not as sensitive as iDES CAPP–Seq, the approach used by Abbosh and colleagues was able to detect ctDNA in 94% of stage I squamous cell carcinoma NSCLC patients. On the other hand, the ctDNA detection rate in patients with adenocarcinoma NSCLC was only 12.8% at stage I, highlighting the interaction between ctDNA detection and cancer (sub-)type.[5,9]

Phallen and colleagues also used a targeted capture approach to detect ctDNA in patients with different cancer types and stages of disease. Their targeted error correction sequencing (TEC–Seq) method utilizes an 81-kb gene panel containing 58 cancer-related genes. Error suppression of their data is based on the start and end position of the reads, as well as a small number of dual-index barcode adapters.[10] Collapsing reads purely based on position is not advised since the size distribution of cirDNA is too tight and different unique molecules could have the same start and end position by chance.[10] Using their general gene panel deep sequencing with 30,000× coverage, Phallen and colleagues were able to detect ctDNA in 62% of all stage I and II patients and 77% of all stage III and IV patients.[10] Similar to the analysis of Bettegowda and colleagues, they also found a difference in detection between different cancer types and an increased detectability with later-stage disease.[9,10]

Recently a method reliant on custom capture sequencing, combined with custom approaches for signal enrichment and sequencing noise suppression, has been used for sensitive detection of ctDNA.[78] This approach, described by Wan and Heider and referred to as INVAR (INtegration of VAriant Reads), targets and integrates signal from hundreds to thousands of patient-specific mutations (as identified by prior sequencing of matched tumour tissue) and has been demonstrated to reliably quantify ctDNA to levels as low as parts per hundred thousand in patients with early-stage lung, kidney,[12] breast, and other cancers.[78] In the case of the former, ctDNA was detected in 12 of 19 patients with stage I–III NSCLC. INVAR also detected stage IV melanoma in 50 of 52 (96%) baseline and follow-up plasma samples.

Alternative Sequencing-Based Methods

Beyond hybrid capture-based approaches, other methods allow for sensitive mutation detection. For example, tagged amplicon deep sequencing (TAm–Seq) is an amplification-based approach that combines singleplex and multiplex amplification steps.[79] Regions of interest are first enriched by amplification in a multiplexed PCR, thereby reducing later sampling bias. The sample is then split and a singleplex PCR of each of the regions of interest is carried out.[79] Amplicons are selected based on publicly available data or cohort-specific knowledge of mutations.[79] The size of the amplicons is around 100 bp, accounting for the majority of cirDNA fragments based on the known distribution of fragment lengths.[15,44] TAm–Seq has a similar sensitivity to dPCR and reduces sampling bias through the first multiplexed amplification step.[80]

Another sequencing-based method is the anchored multiplex PCR (AMP).[81] Initially, designed for the detection of gene rearrangements, this method uses a region-specific forward primer with a universal reverse primer. AMP also detects SNVs, CNVs, insertions, and deletions. Any fragment that contains the sequence corresponding to the forward primer will be amplified and sequenced.[81] This may prove advantageous in the context of ctDNA analysis where the great fragmentation of DNA could lead to a given fragment not covering both primer-binding sites. Using the AMP method, only one primer has to be complementary to a given fragment, thereby increasing the chances of capturing the region of interest.

A recent method, described by Douville and colleagues,[82] uses a single primer to amplify ~350,000 amplicons containing repetitive elements that are evenly distributed throughout the genome. The approach, termed RealSeqS (Repetitive Element Aneuploidy

Sequencing System), was shown to detect aneuploidy in 49% of 883 nonmetastatic cancer patients. Critically, RealSeqS was found to generate meaningful results from as little as 3 pg of input DNA.

McDonald and colleagues developed another sensitive detection method relying on linear pre-amplification followed by single-stranded DNA ligation and multiplex PCR termed targeted digital sequencing (TARDIS).[83] Fragment size information and UMIs are used to suppress errors, resulting in sensitivities of 91% and 53% at allelic fractions of 3 in 10^4 and 3 in 10^5 with a specificity of 96%. TARDIS was applied to stage I–III breast cancer samples and detected ctDNA in all pre-treatment samples and 77% of post-treatment samples.[83]

Lastly, tools like Personalized Analysis of Rearranged Ends (PARE) utilize SVs to detect ctDNA via a PCR-based method.[84] SVs are a common and patient-specific feature among human cancers and are identified through WGS of the tumor sample. Primers covering these unique rearrangement sites can be applied to plasma samples in order to detect ctDNA. PARE is very sensitive since it does not rely on identification of single nucleotide variations (prone to sequencing and PCR errors, as discussed above), but rather on the presence or absence of a PCR product.[84] The major drawback of this method is the need for a tumor sample for initial SV detection, which is not always available.

Summary

Here we have introduced different methods to prepare sequencing libraries from cirDNA samples. One of the most commonly used approaches in the field is double-stranded DNA library preparation. There are a variety of high-quality and easy-to-use kits available, making it a robust method for the preparation of cirDNA samples for sequencing. However, double-stranded library preparations will capture mostly nondegraded fragments longer than 100 bp, thereby not representing all cirDNA populations. Single-stranded DNA library preparation methods have partly addressed this problem by allowing the capture of both shorter and degraded DNA fragments, as well as single- and double-stranded DNAs. However, some of these methods are complex and time consuming while others have shown a bias in fragment incorporation. Both double-stranded and single-stranded DNA library preparation methods contain a PCR step to amplify the cirDNA. Indexing with unique molecular barcodes has been proposed to counteract potential PCR and sequencing biases that arise during the standard preparation process. While indexing will remove a great number of PCR and sequencing errors, they might still fail to correct for early PCR errors or lose data due to PCR and sequencing errors in the barcodes themselves. Recently, PCR-free amplification methods with lower input requirements have been developed, notably for single-cell genomics, making it a feasible alternative to cirDNA sample preparation. The removal of the PCR step results in less-biased sample preparation and eliminates mutations that would otherwise have been induced through PCR errors. Unfortunately, this method requires an input of 50 ng, which is not easily achievable in all cancer settings. We have highlighted the most important advantages and disadvantages of the different library preparation methods in Table 1.

Moreover, we have presented in this chapter various methods for sequencing cirDNA from plasma samples. Figure 2 provides a schematic overview of the preparation process involved in the described methods.

The main difference between the methods is the size of the genome that will be sequenced and the resulting sensitivity, specificity, and sequencing cost per sample. As shown in Fig. 3, the

Table 1. Comparison of Library Preparation Methods

Method	PCR?	Main advantage	Main disadvantage
Double-stranded library preparation[4,48]	Yes	Quick, optimized protocols and low input	Loss of shorter and degraded fragments
Single-strandedlibrary preparation[37,42]	Yes	Low input, capturing short and degraded fragments	Bias in fragment recovery, more complex protocols
Unique molecular identifiers[48,54]	Yes	Reduced noise by read collapsing into consensus sequences	Early PCR errors are missed; sequencing error in UMI sequence incorrectly assigns family members. Greater sequencing depth is required to generate a family of sufficient size for consensus calling
PCR-freelibrary preparation[61]	No	Reduces GC bias, better coverage, no PCR errors	Greater amount of input material needed

methods also differ in the type of somatic event they can detect. While WGS provides the broadest and least biased overview of a given sample, it is also the most expensive if an appreciable depth of sequencing is required. Using capture-based methods, one decreases the window of the genome that is being targeted, thereby reducing the total sequencing cost per sample. Off-the-shelf capture approaches exist that target the whole exome or a cancer specific gene sets. Alternatively, one can design custom capture panels to improve the sequencing of bespoke regions of interest. Lastly, alternative sequencing approaches such as TAm–Seq, RealSeqS, TARDIS, and AMP that can still cover multiple genomic regions were discussed. AMP in particular is an intriguing method since it only requires one site-specific primer, allowing

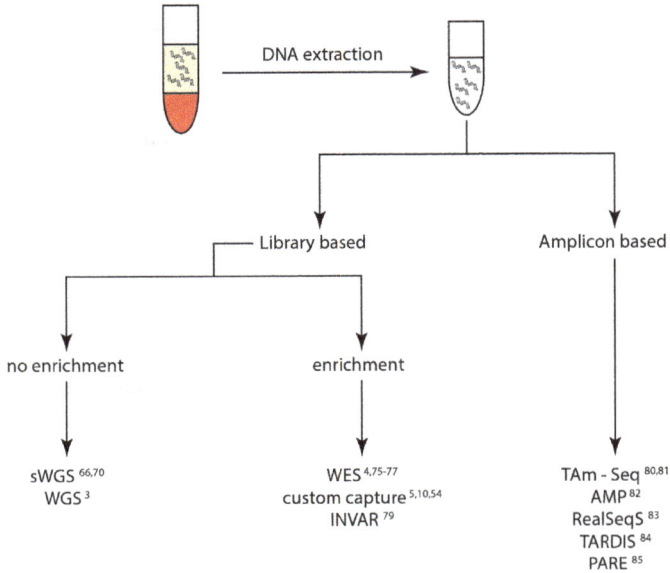

Fig. 2: Overview of preparation process of different cirDNA sequencing methods described in this document.

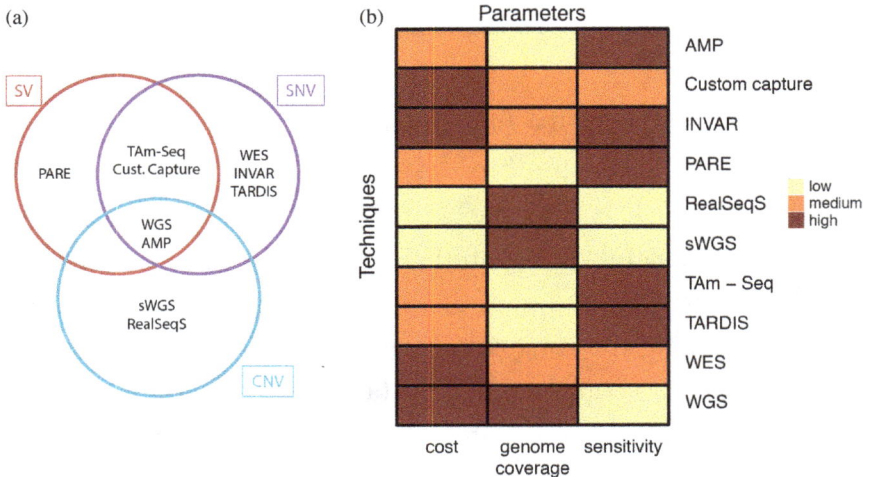

Fig. 3: (a) Overview of described methods for cirDNA analysis. Methods are grouped by variants they can optimally detect (structural variants (SV), single-nucleotide variants (SNV), and copy number variants (CNV)). (b) Methods are compared with respect to cost, sensitivity, and area of the genome covered.

the user to capture fragments of any length as long as they contain the one primer-binding site. Semi-ligated PCR methods, such as AMP, can also be adapted for sensitively detecting new rearrangements in cirDNA.

When choosing the most appropriate sequencing method, it is important to have a good estimation of the expected levels of ctDNA in a given sample. Depending on the ctDNA fraction, more or less sensitive methods will be required for analysis. One potentially useful practice could be to implement sWGS of a given plasma sample prior to choosing the analysis approach. This is because sWGS is a comparatively cheap and rapid technique that can assess likely ctDNA levels. Indeed, the mFast-SeqS and ichorCNA approaches have been demonstrated to aid in determining ctDNA concentration in the plasma, in-turn identifying the best analysis platform.[67,68] These approaches allow the user to group the samples into low and high tumor burden ctDNA samples and, based on this classification, one can then choose an approach for the analysis of the specific alterations in the sample. The only caveat to this would be the reliance on somatic CNVs — this approach would not be as effective in cancers known to carry few somatic CNVs.[26]

Our understanding of cirDNA in the cancer setting and ways to analyze it have improved greatly since it was first described.[85,86] The first diagnostic test using plasma ctDNA to identify NSCLC patients with an *EGFR* exon19 deletion has already been FDA approved for the clinic. This alteration is important as patients carrying this mutation can be effectively treated with the tyrosine kinase inhibitor gefitinib (Iressa).[87] More recently, the COBAS® EGFR mutation test v2 was FDA approved for using plasma samples from NSCLC patients to detect alterations that allow treatment with the tyrosine kinase inhibitors erlotinib (Tarceva) and osimertinib (Tagrisso).[88]

Multiple studies have also shown the utility of ctDNA as a means of identifying recurrence sooner than conventional methods, with important clinical implications.[5,89]

ctDNA has been demonstrated to represent most of the cellular populations that make up a given tumor. As such, it allows a global "snap-shot" of the disease at a given time. Conversely, conventional biopsy techniques might not capture this global representation.[3-5] Additionally, the ease of sampling and minimally invasive nature of cirDNA collection allow for serial monitoring of patients, which would otherwise be harmful using biopsies or CT scans.[6,7] Finally, with the development of easy-to-use kits and the continuous reduction in sequencing costs, the analysis of ctDNA in the clinic represents an increasingly viable and attractive option. Recent developments that tailor sequencing to the biology of ctDNA, innovative sequencing solutions, as well as integration of machine learning analysis of large scale cohorts will also lead to intriguing new avenues for implementation of liquid biopsy in the clinic.

Acknowledgments

The authors would like to thank Nitzan Rosenfeld and all the members of the Rosenfeld group, especially I. Hudecova and D. Gale for proof reading the manuscript. This research was funded by Cancer Research UK (grant numbers A20240), the European Research Council (ERC) under the European Union's Seventh Framework Programme (FP/2007-2013) ERC Grant Agreement number 337905 and supported by the NIHR Cambridge BRC. The views expressed are those of the author(s) and not necessarily those of the NIHR or the Department of Health and Social Care.

References

1. Siravegna G, Marsoni S, Siena S, Bardelli A. (2017) Integrating liquid biopsies into the management of cancer. *Nat Rev Clin Oncol* **14**: 531–548 [http://www.nature.com/doifinder/10.1038/nrclinonc.2017.14]

2. Wan JCM, Massie C, Garcia-Corbacho J, *et al.* (2017) Liquid biopsies come of age: Towards implementation of circulating tumour DNA. *Nat Rev Cancer* **17**: 223–238.

3. Chan KCA, Jiang P, Zheng YWL, *et al.* Cancer genome scanning in plasma: Detection of tumor-associated copy number aberrations, single-nucleotide variants, and tumoral heterogeneity by massively parallel sequencing. *Clin Chem* **59**: 211–224 [http://www.ncbi.nlm.nih.gov/pubmed/23065472]

4. Murtaza M, Dawson S-J, Tsui DWY, *et al.* (2013) Non-invasive analysis of acquired resistance to cancer therapy by sequencing of plasma DNA. *Nature* **497**: 108–112.

5. Abbosh C, Birkbak NJ, Wilson GA, *et al.* (2017) Phylogenetic ctDNA analysis depicts early-stage lung cancer evolution. *Nature* **545**: 446–451.

6. Fazel R, Krumholz HM, Wang Y, *et al.* (2009) Exposure to low-dose ionizing radiation from medical imaging procedures. *N Engl J Med* **361**: 849–857 [http://www.ncbi.nlm.nih.gov/pubmed/19710483]

7. Overman MJ, Modak J, Kopetz S, *et al.* (2013) Use of research biopsies in clinical trials: Are risks and benefits adequately discussed? *J Clin Oncol* **31**: 17–22.

8. Schwarzenbach H, Hoon DSB, Pantel K. (2011) Cell-free nucleic acids as biomarkers in cancer patients. *Nat Rev Cancer* **11**: 426–437 [http://dx.doi.org/10.1038/nrc3066]

9. Bettegowda C, Sausen M, Leary RJ, *et al.* (2014) Detection of circulating tumor DNA in early-and late-stage human malignancies. *Sci Transl Med* **6**: 224ra24–224ra24 [http://stm.sciencemag.org/cgi/doi/10.1126/scitranslmed.3007094]

10. Phallen J, Sausen M, Adleff V, *et al.* (2017) Direct detection of early-stage cancers using circulating tumor DNA. *Sci Transl Med* **9**: eaan2415.

11. Mouliere F, Chandrananda D, Piskorz AM, *et al.* (2018) Enhanced detection of circulating tumor DNA by fragment size analysis. *Sci Transl Med* **10**: eaat4921.

12. Smith CG, Moser T, Mouliere F, *et al.* (2020) Comprehensive characterization of cell-free tumor DNA in plasma and urine of patients with renal tumors. *Genome Med* **12**(1): 23.

13. Jahr S, Hentze H, Englisch S, *et al.* (2001) DNA fragments in the blood plasma of cancer patients: Quantitations and evidence for their origin from apoptotic and necrotic cells. *Cancer Res* **61**: 1659–1665.

14. Parkinson CA, Gale D, Piskorz AM, *et al.* (2016) Exploratory analysis of TP53 mutations in circulating tumour DNA as biomarkers of treatment response for patients with relapsed high-grade serous ovarian carcinoma: A retrospective study. Mardis ER, editor. *PLOS Med* **13**: e1002198.

15. Lo YMD, Chan KCA, Sun H, *et al.* (2010) Maternal plasma DNA sequencing reveals the genome-wide genetic and mutational profile of the fetus. *Sci Transl Med* 2010 Dec 8; **2**(61): 61ra91 [http://stm.sciencemag.org/content/2/61/61ra91.full]

16. Chandrananda D, Thorne NP, Bahlo M. (2015) High-resolution characterization of sequence signatures due to non-random cleavage of cell-free DNA. *BMC Med Genomics* **8**: 29 [http://bmcmedgenomics.biomedcentral.com/articles/10.1186/s12920-015-0107-z]

17. Lichtenstein AV, Melkonyan HS, Tomei LD, Umansky SR. (2001) Circulating nucleic acids and apoptosis. *Ann N Y Acad Sci* **945**: 239–249 [http://www.ncbi.nlm.nih.gov/pubmed/11708486]

18. Mouliere F, Robert B, Arnau Peyrotte E, *et al.* (2011) High fragmentation characterizes tumour-derived circulating DNA. Lee T, editor. *PLOS One* **6**: e23418 [http://dx.plos.org/10.1371/journal.pone.0023418]

19. Underhill HR, Kitzman JO, Hellwig S, *et al.* (2016) Fragment length of circulating tumor DNA. *PLOS Genet* 2016 Jul 18;**12**(7): e1006162

20. Jiang P, Sun K, Peng W, *et al.* (2020) Plasma DNA end-motif profiling as a fragmentomic marker in cancer, pregnancy, and transplantation. *Cancer Discov* **10**: 664–673 [https://pubmed.ncbi.nlm.nih.gov/32111602/]

21. Shendure J, Ji H. (2008) Next-generation DNA sequencing. *Nat Biotechnol* **26**: 1135–1145 [http://www.nature.com/doifinder/10.1038/nbt1486]

22. Valle-Inclan JE, Stangl C, de Jong AC, *et al.* (2021) Optimizing nanopore sequencing-based detection of structural variants enables individualized circulating tumor DNA-based disease monitoring in cancer patients. *Genome*

Med **13**: 86 [https://genomemedicine.biomedcentral.com/articles/10.1186/s13073-021-00899-7]

23. Urosevic N, Inglis TJJ, Grasko J, Lim EM. (2013) Evaluation of clinical laboratory methods for plasma cell-Free DNA analysis in suspected septicaemia. *J Med Diagn Meth* **2**(3) [https://www.omicsgroup.org/journals/evaluation-of-clinical-laboratory-methods-for-plasma-cell-free-dna-analysis-in-suspected-septicaemia-2168-9784.1000123.php?aid=17035]

24. Ponti G, Maccaferri M, Manfredini M, *et al.* The value of fluorimetry (Qubit) and spectrophotometry (NanoDrop) in the quantification of cell-free DNA (cfDNA) in malignant melanoma and prostate cancer patients. *Clin Chim Acta* **479**: 14–19 [http://linkinghub.elsevier.com/retrieve/pii/S000989811830007X]

25. Vogelstein B, Kinzler KW. (1999) Digital PCR. *Proc Natl Acad Sci USA* **96**: 9236–9241 [http://www.ncbi.nlm.nih.gov/pubmed/10430926]

26. Ciriello G, Miller ML, Aksoy BA, Senbabaoglu Y, Schultz N, Sander C. (2013) Emerging landscape of oncogenic signatures across human cancers. *Nat Genet* **45**: 1127–1133 [http://www.nature.com/doifinder/10.1038/ng.2762]

27. Devonshire AS, Whale AS, Gutteridge A, *et al.* (2014) Towards standardisation of cell-free DNA measurement in plasma: Controls for extraction efficiency, fragment size bias and quantification. *Anal Bioanal Chem* **406**: 6499–6512 [http://www.ncbi.nlm.nih.gov/pubmed/24853859]

28. Linnarsson S. (2010) Recent advances in DNA sequencing methods — general principles of sample preparation. *Exp Cell Res* **316**: 1339–1343 [http://www.sciencedirect.com/science/article/pii/S0014482710000984]

29. Head SR, Komori HK, LaMere SA, *et al.* (2014) Library construction for next-generation sequencing: Overviews and challenges. *Biotechniques* **56**: 61–64, 66, 68, passim [http://www.ncbi.nlm.nih.gov/pubmed/24502796]

30. Van Dijk EL, Jaszczszyn Y, Thermes C. (2014) Library preparation methods for next-generation sequencing: Tone down the bias. *Exp Cell Res* **322**: 12–20.

31. Malapelle U, Pisapia P, Rocco D, *et al.* (2016) Next generation sequencing techniques in liquid biopsy: Focus on non-small cell lung cancer patients. *Transl Lung Cancer Res* **5**: 505–510 [http://www.ncbi.nlm.nih.gov/pubmed/27826531]

32. Quail MA, Kozarewa I, Smith F, *et al.* (2008) A large genome center's improvements to the Illumina sequencing system. *Nat Methods* **5**: 1005–1010 [http://www.nature.com/doifinder/10.1038/nmeth.1270]

33. van Dijk EL, Auger H, Jaszczyszyn Y, Thermes C. (2014) Ten years of next-generation sequencing technology. *Trends Genet* **30**: 418–426 [http://www.sciencedirect.com/science/article/pii/S0168952514001127?via%3Dihub]

34. Burnham P, Kim MS, Agbor-Enoh S, *et al.* (2016) Single-stranded DNA library preparation uncovers the origin and diversity of ultrashort cell-free DNA in plasma. *Sci Rep* **6**: 27859 [http://www.nature.com/articles/srep27859]

35. Gansauge M-T, Meyer M. (2013) Single-stranded DNA library preparation for the sequencing of ancient or damaged DNA. *Nat Protoc* **8**: 737–748 [http://www.nature.com/doifinder/10.1038/nprot.2013.038]

36. Snyder MW, Kircher M, Hill AJ, Daza RM, Shendure J. (2016) Cell-free DNA comprises an in vivo nucleosome footprint that informs its tissues-of-origin. *Cell* **164**: 57–68.

37. Gansauge M-T, Gerber T, Glocke I, *et al.* (2017) Single-stranded DNA library preparation from highly degraded DNA using T4 DNA ligase. *Nucleic Acids Res* **45**: e79 [http://www.ncbi.nlm.nih.gov/pubmed/28119419]

38. Mouliere F, Rosenfeld N. (2015) Circulating tumor-derived DNA is shorter than somatic DNA in plasma. *Proc Natl Acad Sci* **112**: 3178–3179.

39. Jiang P, Chan CWM, Chan KCA, *et al.* (2015) Lengthening and shortening of plasma DNA in hepatocellular carcinoma patients. *Proc Natl Acad Sci* **112**: E1317–E1325.

40. Moser T, Ulz P, Zhou Q, *et al.* (2017) Single-stranded DNA library preparation does not preferentially enrich circulating tumor DNA. *Clin Chem* **63**: 1656–1659 [http://clinchem.aaccjnls.org/content/early/2017/08/07/clinchem.2017.277988.long]

41. Zhu YY, Machleder EM, Chenchik A, Li R, Siebert PD. (2001) Reverse transcriptase template switching: A SMART approach for full-length cDNA library construction. *Biotechniques* **30**: 892–897 [http://www.ncbi.nlm.nih.gov/pubmed/11314272]

42. Turchinovich A, Surowy H, Serva A, Zapatka M, Lichter P, Burwinkel B. (2014) Capture and amplification by tailing and switching (CATS). An ultrasensitive ligation-independent method for generation of DNA librar-

ies for deep sequencing from picogram amounts of DNA and RNA. *RNA Biol* **11**: 817–828 [http://www.ncbi.nlm.nih.gov/pubmed/24922482]

43. Vardi O, Shamir I, Javasky E, Goren A, Simon I. (2017) Biases in the SMART-DNA library preparation method associated with genomic poly dA/dT sequences. Bandapalli OR, editor. *PLOS ONE* **12**: e0172769 [http://dx.plos.org/10.1371/journal.pone.0172769]

44. Thierry AR, Mouliere F, Gongora C, *et al.* (2010) Origin and quantification of circulating DNA in mice with human colorectal cancer xenografts. *Nucleic Acids Res* **38**: 6159–6175 [https://academic.oup.com/nar/article-lookup/doi/10.1093/nar/gkq421]

45. Mouliere F, Piskorz AM, Chandrananda D, *et al.* (2017) Selecting short DNA fragments in plasma improves detection of circulating tumour DNA. *bioRxiv*: 134437.

46. Song P, Chen SX, Yan YH, *et al.* (2021) Selective multiplexed enrichment for the detection and quantitation of low-fraction DNA variants via low-depth sequencing. *Nat Biomed Eng* **5**(7): 690–701 [https://pubmed.ncbi.nlm.nih.gov/33941896/]

47. Lou DI, Hussmann JA, McBee RM, *et al.* (2013) High-throughput DNA sequencing errors are reduced by orders of magnitude using circle sequencing. *Proc Natl Acad Sci* **110**: 19872–19877 [http://www.ncbi.nlm.nih.gov/pubmed/24243955]

48. Kinde I, Wu J, Papadopoulos N, Kinzler KW, Vogelstein B. (2011) Detection and quantification of rare mutations with massively parallel sequencing. *Proc Natl Acad Sci U S A* **108**: 9530–9535 [http://www.ncbi.nlm.nih.gov/pubmed/21586637]

49. Robin JD, Ludlow AT, LaRanger R, Wright WE, Shay JW. (2016) Comparison of DNA quantification methods for next generation sequencing. *Sci Rep* **6**: 24067 [http://www.nature.com/articles/srep24067]

50. Hug H, Schuler R. (2003) Measurement of the number of molecules of a single mRNA species in a complex mRNA preparation. *J Theor Biol* **221**: 615–624 [http://www.ncbi.nlm.nih.gov/pubmed/12713944]

51. Casbon JA, Osborne RJ, Brenner S, Lichtenstein CP. (2011) A method for counting PCR template molecules with application to next-generation sequencing. *Nucleic Acids Res* **39**: e81–e81 [https://academic.oup.com/nar/article-lookup/doi/10.1093/nar/gkr217]

52. Kou R, Lam H, Duan H, *et al.* (2016) Benefits and challenges with applying unique molecular identifiers in next generation sequencing to detect low frequency mutations. Wang J, editor. *PLOS ONE* **11**: e0146638 [http://dx.plos.org/10.1371/journal.pone.0146638]

53. Smith T, Heger A, Sudbery I. (2017) UMI-tools: Modeling sequencing errors in unique molecular Identifiers to improve quantification accuracy. *Genome Res* **27**: 491–499 [http://www.ncbi.nlm.nih.gov/pubmed/28100584]

54. Newman AM, Lovejoy AF, Klass DM, *et al.* (2016) Integrated digital error suppression for improved detection of circulating tumor DNA. *Nat Biotechnol* **34**: 547–555.

55. Perakis S, Speicher MR. (2017) Emerging concepts in liquid biopsies. *BMC Med* **15**: 75 [http://www.ncbi.nlm.nih.gov/pubmed/28381299]

56. UM BRCF Bioinformatics Core. (2017) *CONNOR* [https://github.com/umich-brcf-bioinf/Connor]

57. Shugay M, Zaretsky AR, Shagin DA, *et al.* (2017) MAGERI: Computational pipeline for molecular-barcoded targeted resequencing. Gardner PP, editor. *PLOS Comput Biol* **13**: e1005480 [http://dx.plos.org/10.1371/journal.pcbi.1005480]

58. Agilent. (2017) *SureCall* [https://www.genomics.agilent.com/en/NGS-Data-Analysis-Software/SureCall/?cid=AG-PT-154&tabId=AG-PR-1196]

59. Schmitt MW, Kennedy SR, Salk JJ, Fox EJ, Hiatt JB, Loeb LA. (2012) Detection of ultra-rare mutations by next-generation sequencing. *Proc Natl Acad Sci U S A* **109**: 14508–14513 [http://www.ncbi.nlm.nih.gov/pubmed/22853953]

60. Cohen JD, Douville C, Dudley JC, *et al.* (2021) Detection of low-frequency DNA variants by targeted sequencing of the Watson and Crick strands. *Nat Biotechnol* **39**(10):1220–1227.

61. Karlsson K, Sahlin E, Iwarsson E, Westgren M, Nordenskjöld M, Linnarsson S. (2015) Amplification-free sequencing of cell-free DNA for prenatal non-invasive diagnosis of chromosomal aberrations. *Genomics* **105**: 150–158 [http://www.ncbi.nlm.nih.gov/pubmed/25543032]

62. Dean FB, Hosono S, Fang L, *et al.* (2002) Comprehensive human genome amplification using multiple displacement amplification. *Proc Natl Acad Sci U S A* **99**: 5261–5266 [http://www.ncbi.nlm.nih.gov/pubmed/11959976]

63. Goodwin S, McPherson JD, McCombie WR. (2016) Coming of age: Ten years of next-generation sequencing technologies. *Nat Rev Genet* **17**: 333–351 [schatz]

64. Wang T-L, Maierhofer C, Speicher MR, *et al.* (2002) Digital karyotyping. *Proc Natl Acad Sci U S A* **99**: 16156–16161 [http://www.ncbi.nlm.nih.gov/pubmed/12461184]

65. Leary RJ, Sausen M, Kinde I, *et al.* (2012) Detection of chromosomal alterations in the circulation of cancer patients with whole-genome sequencing. *Sci Transl Med* **4**: 162ra154 [http://www.ncbi.nlm.nih.gov/pubmed/23197571]

66. Hanahan D, Weinberg RA. (2000) The hallmarks of cancer. *Cell* **100**: 57–70 [http://linkinghub.elsevier.com/retrieve/pii/S0092867400816839]

67. Adalsteinsson VA, Ha G, Freeman SS, *et al.* (2017) Scalable whole-exome sequencing of cell-free DNA reveals high concordance with metastatic tumors. *Nat Commun* **8**: 1324.

68. Belic J, Koch M, Ulz P, *et al.* (2015) Rapid identification of plasma DNA samples with increased ctDNA levels by a modified FAST-SeqS approach. *Clin Chem* **61**: 838–849.

69. Heitzer E, Ulz P, Belic J, *et al.* (2013) Tumor-associated copy number changes in the circulation of patients with prostate cancer identified through whole-genome sequencing. *Genome Med* **5**: 30 [http://genomemedicine.biomedcentral.com/articles/10.1186/gm434]

70. Cristiano S, Leal A, Phallen J, *et al.* (2019) Genome-wide cell-free DNA fragmentation in patients with cancer. *Nature* 570(7761): 385–389 [http://www.nature.com/articles/s41586-019-1272-6]

71. Zviran A, Schulman RC, Shah M, *et al.* (2020) Genome-wide cell-free DNA mutational integration enables ultra-sensitive cancer monitoring. *Nat Med* **26**: 1114–1124.

72. Genohub. (2015) *Whole Genome Sequencing (WGS) vs. Whole Exome Sequencing (WES)* [https://blog.genohub.com/2015/02/21/whole-genome-sequencing-wgs-vs-whole-exome-sequencing-wes/]

73. Samorodnitsky E, Jewell BM, Hagopian R, *et al.* (2015) Evaluation of hybridization capture versus amplicon-based methods for whole-exome sequencing. *Hum Mutat* **36**: 903–914 [http://www.ncbi.nlm.nih.gov/pubmed/26110913]

74. Girotti MR, Gremel G, Lee R, *et al.* (2016) Application of sequencing, liquid biopsies, and patient-derived xenografts for personalized medicine in melanoma. *Cancer Discov* **6**: 286–299.

75. Dietz S, Schirmer U, Mercé C, *et al.* (2016) Low input whole-exome sequencing to determine the representation of the tumor exome in circulating DNA of non-small cell lung cancer patients. *PLOS ONE* **11**: e0161012 [http://www.ncbi.nlm.nih.gov/pubmed/27529345]

76. Butler TM, Johnson-Camacho K, Peto M, *et al.* (2015) Exome sequencing of cell-free DNA from metastatic cancer patients identifies clinically actionable mutations distinct from primary disease. Richards KL, editor. *PLOS ONE* **10**: e0136407 [http://dx.plos.org/10.1371/journal.pone.0136407]

77. Newman AM, Bratman S V, To J, *et al.* (2014) An ultrasensitive method for quantitating circulating tumor DNA with broad patient coverage. *Nat Med* **20**: 548–554 [http://www.ncbi.nlm.nih.gov/pubmed/24705333]

78. Wan JCM, Heider K, Gale D, *et al.* (2020) ctDNA monitoring using patient-specific sequencing and integration of variant reads. *Sci Transl Med* **12**: eaaz8084.

79. Forshew T, Murtaza M, Parkinson C, *et al.* (2012) Noninvasive identification and monitoring of cancer mutations by targeted deep sequencing of plasma DNA. *Sci Transl Med* **4**: 136ra68–136ra68.

80. Dawson S-J, Tsui DWY, Murtaza M, *et al.* (2013) Analysis of circulating tumor DNA to monitor metastatic breast cancer. *N Engl J Med* **368**: 1199–1209.

81. Zheng Z, Liebers M, Zhelyazkova B, *et al.* (2014) Anchored multiplex PCR for targeted next-generation sequencing. *Nat Med* **20**: 1479–1484 [http://www.nature.com/doifinder/10.1038/nm.3729]

82. Douville C, Cohen JD, Ptak J, *et al.* Assessing aneuploidy with repetitive element sequencing. Proc Natl Acad Sci U S A 2020 Mar 3; **117**(9): 4858–4863. doi: 10.1073/pnas.1910041117. Epub 2020 Feb 19.

83. McDonald BR, Contente-Cuomo T, Sammut S-J, *et al.* (2019) Personalized circulating tumor DNA analysis to detect residual disease after neoadjuvant therapy in breast cancer. *Sci Transl Med* **11**: eaax7392 [http://stm.sciencemag.org/lookup/doi/10.1126/scitranslmed.aax7392]

84. Leary RJ, Kinde I, Diehl F, *et al.* (2010) Development of personalized tumor biomarkers using massively parallel sequencing. *Sci Transl Med* **2**: 20ra14 [http://www.ncbi.nlm.nih.gov/pubmed/20371490]

85. Leon SA, Shapiro B, Sklaroff DM, Yaros MJ. (1977) Free DNA in the serum of cancer patients and the effect of therapy. *Cancer Res* **37**: 646–650 [http://www.ncbi.nlm.nih.gov/pubmed/837366]

86. Stroun M, Anker P, Lyautey J, Lederrey C, Maurice PA. (1987) Isolation and characterization of DNA from the plasma of cancer patients. *Eur J Cancer Clin Oncol* **23**: 707–712 [https://www.sciencedirect.com/science/article/pii/0277537987902665]

87. European Medicines Agency. (2014) *Iressa: EPAR-Product Information* [http://www.ema.europa.eu/docs/en_GB/document_library/EPAR_-_Product_Information/human/001016/WC500036358.pdf]

88. FDA. (2016) *cobas® EGFR Mutation Test v2 approval* [https://www.accessdata.fda.gov/cdrh_docs/pdf15/P150044A.pdf]

89. Pereira E, Camacho-Vanegas O, Anand S, *et al.* (2015) Personalized circulating tumor DNA biomarkers dynamically predict treatment response and survival in gynecologic cancers. *PLOS ONE* **10**: e0145754 [http://dx.plos.org/10.1371/journal.pone.0145754]

Chapter 7

Blood Nucleases Affecting Circulating DNA in Serum and Plasma

Gustavo Barra

Abstract

Circulating cell-free DNA (cirDNA) is extracellular DNA occurring in the blood.[1] It is a biomarker of growing interest in various clinical fields, especially in prenatal diagnosis and oncology, because it allows sampling of fetal or tumor DNA while avoiding the risks associated with invasive tissue biopsies. The existence of a DNA-degrading activity in the blood is also well established; however, the impact of these enzymes as a preanalytical variable in cirDNA assays and studies have been long neglected. The significance of blood DNAses is 2-fold. Firstly, they are intimately involved in the physiological mechanisms of cirDNA generation and clearance and as such are responsible for the size profile, cleavage patterns, and concentration of cirDNA in blood. Secondly, the activity of blood DNAses in plasma and serum after sample collection contributes to experimental artifacts including decreasing DNA concentration, changing size distribution, and DNA sequences of interest falling below detectable levels. A detailed understanding of DNases biological properties is essential to making the best use of cirDNA in different clinical settings. Thus, this chapter is a review of the types, functions, biology, and clinical correlates for the DNases found in the circulation. Moreover, it contains a summary of the main results observed by our research group about the blood DNase ex vivo effect over the cirDNA in the most commonly used cell-free samples.

Biological Role of Blood DNases

Unprotected exogenous single-stranded oligonucleotides and double-stranded DNA are rapidly degraded in vitro[2-4] and in vivo[5,6] suggesting that protection against foreign nucleic acids is one of blood DNases' biological roles.[7] A role in the prevention of horizontal transfer of gene sequences from one cell to another can also be speculated.[8] Similarly, these enzymes degrade endogenous nucleic acids that appear in the circulation as consequence of DNA released by living, apoptotic and necrotic cells, as well as by other mechanisms (e.g., NETosis), maintaining the physiological level of DNA in the circulation.[9]

An inverse correlation between the cirDNA yield and blood DNase activity has been reported[10,11] and failure of the DNA clearance mechanism has been involved in pathogenesis of autoimmune diseases (e.g., systemic lupus erythematosus).[12-14] For example, serum DNAse I, C1q[15] and factor VII-activating protease[16] cooperate in the degradation of chromatin and removal of dying cells by macrophages, which is essential for tissue homeostasis and resolution of inflammation.[17]

Howsoever, DNases do not seem to be the major mechanism for cirDNA removal from the bloodstream.[18,19] In addition to its breakdown by DNases, intake by cells,[8] liver,[8] and kidney[20] metabolism can clear cirDNA. The association of the DNA with

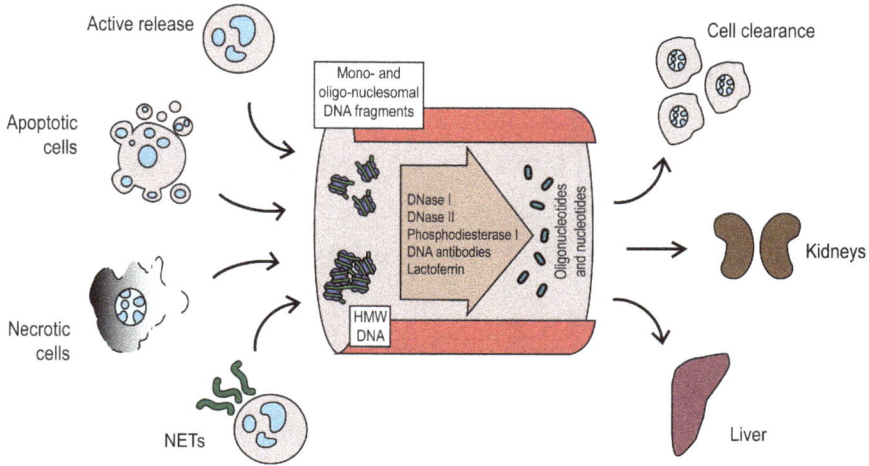

Fig. 1: Sources of cirDNA and physiological clearance mechanism.

nucleosomes seems to have an important effect on the uptake and breakdown processes.[8]

In spite of the clearance mechanism, fetal cirDNA has a mean half-life of only 16.3 min in maternal plasma[19] and tumor cirDNA in the blood has a half-life of ~2 hr.[21] This evidence suggests that cirDNA elimination from blood is fast, and a continuous supply is necessary to maintain a specific cirDNA sequence at a constant level in the circulation (Fig. 1).

Role of DNases in cirDNA Origins

cirDNA is fragmented, occurring mainly as short, but also as long, double-stranded molecules. Thus, it is generated by mechanisms that involve the action of DNases. Understanding which enzymes are involved in its origins would contribute to making the best use of these molecules. In this section, a connection between cirDNA fragment size and the DNases that generate such fragment patterns will be discussed.

cirDNA Origin

Recent studies have shown that majority of cirDNA in healthy individuals originates from hematopoietic cell death and it is a heterogeneous mixture of sequences from lymphoid and myeloid cell types.[22] CirDNA yields ladder-like banding patterns equivalent to whole-number multiples of the ~170 bp nucleosomal unit DNA in gel electrophoresis,[23,24] which is similar to the pattern observed in degraded DNA from apoptotic cells[25] suggesting that cirDNA originates from cell dying by this process. Indeed, apoptosis is a common, critical, and actively regulated process during hematopoiesis and in mature hematopoietic cell types.[26] Additionally, nondividing cells, such as lymphocytes, and cultured cell lines including HL-60 spontaneously release a nucleoprotein complex within a homeostatic system in which newly synthetized DNA is preferentially released.[27] This spontaneously released DNA also has a ladder-like banding pattern in gel electrophoresis. Larger DNA molecules (>10,000 bp) have also been observed in cirDNA and such molecules are speculated to come from cells dying via necrosis.[28] DNA released by necrosis is incompletely and nonspecifically digested and thus smears on electrophoretic separation due to its larger fragment sizes.[27]

In nonphysiological conditions such as cancer or acute/chronic tissue damage there is additional sequence contribution from one or more nonhematopoietic cell types to the cirDNA pool. These additional sequences, as well as the aberrant contribution from hematopoietic cell lineages, have tremendous potential as a "liquid biopsy."[22] However, the relative contribution of each above-cited processes to the cirDNA levels in pathological conditions (e.g., myocardial infarction, stroke, autoimmune disorders and cancer) is still under investigation.

Finally, NETosis is another mechanism that may produce cirDNA in pathological conditions. Upon activation, neutrophils (the most abundant population of white blood cells) can release extracellular nucleic acids decorated with histones and granular proteins capable of entrapping pathogens.[29] These DNA structures, named neutrophil extracellular traps (NETs), can be formed within blood vessels[30] (Fig. 1).

cirDNA Fragment Size

Advanced technologies of massively parallel sequencing have provided unprecedented opportunities to investigate the size profile of cirDNA.[31] The distribution of fragment lengths of cirDNA is multimodal. The most prominent peak was around ~167 bp, with next occurring at ~340 bp. A much wider mode is observed around ~510 bp. These three peaks appear to correspond to the lengths of DNA associated with a mono-, di-, and tri-nucleosome structure, respectively.[32] While the first cell-free DNA mode peaks at ~167 bp, it is preceded by a series of smaller peaks occurring at approximately 10 bp periodicity below ~145 bp (~145, ~134, ~123, ~113, ~102, ~92, and ~82 bp).[32,33] Moreover, minute quantities (0.06%--0.3%) of sequences larger than 1000 bp have been observed.[34] This adds evidence to the hypothesis that the nucleosome packaging and the approximately 10 bp 360° turn of the double helix are key determinants for the fragmentation of the cirDNA.[32]

DNA Degradation During Apoptosis

Firstly the chromosomal DNA is cleaved into large fragments of 50–300 kB (a size consistent with chromatin loop domains[8]) by topoisomerase II,[35] apoptosis-inducing factor,[36] and/or caspase activated DNase (CAD).[37] Subsequently, CAD (caspase-dependent apoptotic pathway)[38,39] or endonuclease G[40] DNase γ and DNase I[41] (caspase-independent apoptotic pathway) cleave these large DNA fragments in oligonucleosomes and/or mononucleosomes.[42] Then, after the apoptotic cells are engulfed by macrophages, DNase II further degrades the fragmented DNA in their lysosomes.[43] Given the high cellular turnover and/or saturation of the mechanism, it is not surprising that some DNAs escape final cleavage/degradation and thus appear in the circulation.[44]

DNA Protection by Nucleosome Structure

The core particle of a nucleosome consists of an octamer of two copies of the four histones H2A, H2B, H3, and H4 — around which ~146 bp of helical DNA is wrapped.[8] An additional ~20 bp should be added if the DNA connected to the peripheral histone H1 is considered (~165 bp).[32] Negatively charged DNA is electrostatically bound to the positively charged histones and individual mononucleosomes are connected by a stretch of linker DNA.[45] During apoptosis, DNases cleave linker DNA more easily than nucleosome-bound DNA, thus resulting in the classic ladder pattern of fragment sizes associated with programmed cell death.[46]

DNases that Cleave the DNA within the Nucleosome Core

As detailed below, DNase I can cut within and outside nucleosomal DNA generating a cleavage signature of 10.3 base oscillation that corresponds to the accessibility of the minor groove as DNA winds around the nucleosome. A similar nick pattern is observed for Endonuclease G but not for CAD.

Blood DNases and the cirDNA Cleavage Signature

The fragment size profile described above suggests that cirDNA fragments are derived from the enzymatic processing of DNA from apoptotic cells.[33] However, DNase I (the main nuclease found in blood) generates similar DNA cleavage patterns and cannot be excluded as a player in the process that generates the observed cleavage signature. Thus, it is possible that, independent of the mechanisms that may produce cirDNA (apoptosis, necrosis, active release, and netosis), blood DNases shape its size pattern. In conclusion, cellular DNases and/or blood DNases together with the protection conferred by nucleosome packing are likely to be the key determinants for cirDNA fragment size distribution observed in the blood.

Types of DNAses

DNases are enzymes capable of hydrolyzing the most stable chemical bond found in biological molecules, the phosphodiester bond.[47] Enzymes capable of degrading DNA in the human blood are deoxyribonuclease I, deoxyribonuclease II, phosphodiesterase I, DNA-hydrolyzing antibodies, and lactoferrin. Some of their characteristics will be detailed in the following and a summary can be found in Table 1. The DNases involved in apoptosis will also be addressed in this section and are summarized in Table 2.

DNAses in Blood

Deoxyribonuclease I (DNAse I)

Deoxyribonuclease I is responsible for 90% of the DNase activity of blood.[48] It is characterized by neutral pH optimum, bivalent

Table 1.   Characteristics of the DNAses Found in Blood

DNases	Concentration	Preferred substrate	Bivalent ions	EDTA
DNAse I	High	dsDNA>>ssDNA	Dependent	Inhibited
DNAse II	Low	dsDNA>>ssDNA	Independent	Not inhibited
Phosphodiesterase I	Low	ssDNA, RNA>>dsDNA	Dependent	Inhibited
DNA-hydrolyzing antibodies	Low	dsDNA>>ssDNA	Dependent	Inhibited
Lactoferrin	Low	dsDNA>>ssDNA	Stimulated	Inhibited

Table 2.   Characteristics of the DNAses Involved in Apoptosis

DNases	Location	Preferred substrate	Bivalent ions	EDTA
Caspase-activated DNase	Nuclei/ cytoplasm	dsDNA	Dependent	Inhibited
Endonuclease G	Mitochondria	ssDNA, RNA>>dsDNA	Dependent	Inhibited
DNAse γ	Nuclei	ssDNA>>dsDNA	Dependent	Inhibited
L-DNase II	Cytoplasm	dsDNA>>ssDNA	Independent	Not inhibited

metal ion (Ca^{2+} and Mg^{2+}) requirement for catalytic activity,[49] and formation of oligonucleotides and nucleotides with a hydroxyl group at the 3′-end and a phosphate group at the 5′-end.[50] DNase I is 100–500 times more active in hydrolysis of double-stranded DNA than of single-stranded.[51] The enzyme binds only with the DNA minor groove,[52,53] interacts with both DNA strands,[51] and introduces one to several single-strand breaks into both strands, which are shifted by several nucleotides.[54] DNase I digests with a ~10 bp periodicity around nucleosomes matching the exposure of the DNA minor groove as it wraps around histones.[55,56]

DNAse I is a secretory protein.[7] Pancreas and parotid glands are the enzyme's major sources, consistent with its role in digesting nucleic acids in the gastrointestinal tract.[57] It is also found in kidney, urine, blood, and seminal fluid, suggesting additional functions.[48] A significant portion of blood DNAse I has pancreatic origin; other sources include the pituitary.[7] The concentration of active DNAse I level in blood measured by single radial enzyme-diffusion assay is 65 ± 27 units/mg protein, a value corresponding to 4.4 units/L.[48] For comparison, its level in urine is $6000 ± 2000 \times 10^3$ units/mg protein.[48] In blood, the analysis of catalytic activity is more appropriate than the analysis of enzyme concentration,[58] because the proportion of the active form is influenced by the presence of the enzyme's natural inhibitor, actin.[59]

Deoxyribonuclease II (DNAse II)

Human DNase II is characterized by acidic pH optimum, lack of bivalent ion (Ca^{2+} and Mg^{2+}) requirement, and formation of DNA reaction products with a hydroxyl group at the 5′-end and a phosphate group at the 3′-end.[60] It is 5–10 times more active on double-stranded DNA than on single-stranded and cannot hydrolyze RNA.[61] Similarly to DNase I, DNAse II hydrolyses the phosphodiester backbone by single-strand nicks rather than double-strand cuts.[60,62] The enzyme is found in the lysosomes of almost all human cells and is believed to be involved in intracellular breakdown of DNA.[7,60] Its activity is also found in saliva, blood, urine, and seminal liquid.[7] Human blood is characterized by low content of DNAse II activity, 0.11 ± 0.009 units/mg protein.[58] Finally, since DNase II has no divalent cation requirement, it is insensitive to the chelating agent EDTA.[62]

Phosphodiesterase I

Members of the phosphodiesterase I family have alkaline pH optimum, require bivalent metal ions (Ca^{2+}, Zn^{2+} and Mg^{2+}) for catalytic activity, and remove 5′-mononucleotides successively from the 3′-hydroxy termini of both DNA and RNA.[63,64] There is evidence that these enzymes show preference for single-stranded or denatured substrates.[65,66] The membrane form of phosphodiesterase I is one of the key enzymes responsible for degradation of nucleic acid fragments to nucleosides.[67] Hydrolyzing foreign DNA and RNA, this enzyme plays a protective role.[7] Family members have been found in the kidney, pancreas, uterus, liver, and heart, and in the following body fluids: seminal liquid, serum, bile, urine, milk, and cerebrospinal liquid.[7,68] The normal values in human blood serum were determined to be 33 ± 6.4 units/L by a phosphodiesterase activity assay[68] and 36 ng/mL by ELISA.[69] EDTA totally inhibits the catalytic activity of phosphodiesterase I.[68,70]

DNA-Hydrolyzing Antibodies

Autoantibodies with DNA-nicking activity have been detected in the serum of patients with autoimmune diseases (e.g., systemic lupus erythematous,[71] multiple sclerosis,[72] and others[7]). Their effectiveness of hydrolysis of double-stranded DNA is 3–5 times higher than single-stranded.[73] The DNA-nicking activity is dependent on metal ions (Mg^{2+}, Mn^{2+}, and Ca^{2+}) and is inhibited by EDTA.[71] The cleavage patterns of DNA-hydrolyzing antibodies do not have any cleavage-site specificity and differ from those produced by DNAse from human serum and DNAse I.[71] Their activity in patient serum is two orders of magnitude less than that of DNAse I[71] and is not detected or negligible in healthy subjects.[71,72]

Lactoferrin

Lactoferrin is a unique polyfunctional protein and possesses five different catalytic activities: RNase, DNase, phosphatase,

ATPase, and amylase.[7] The enzyme is more effective in cleavage of double-strand DNA than that of oligonucleotides, has maximal activity at neutral pH, and is stimulated by bivalent ions (Cu^{2+}, Zn^{2+}, Ca^{2+}, Mg^{2+}, and Mn^{2+}). EDTA at concentrations of 10 mM or higher inhibited its activity.[74] Lactoferrin is the major nuclease of human milk[74] and has been found in a wide range of other human external secretion (saliva, tears, urine, and others)[75] as well as in the specific granules of neutrophilic leukocytes.[76] The enzyme is present in blood at a very low concentration and its level appears correlated to the neutrophil turnover.[77] In healthy subjects, the lactoferrin level in plasma is 168 ± 100 µg/L (imunoenzymatic assay) and its concentration is slightly higher in serum (237 ± 155 µg/L),[78] probably because of neutrophil lysis during coagulation.[79]

Intracellular DNases Involved in the Apoptosis

Two classes of nucleases degrade the cellular DNA during apoptosis: (a) the cell autonomous nucleases (e.g., CAD and Endo G), which cleave DNA within the dying cell and are responsible for DNA laddering; and (b) the cell nonautonomous nucleases (e.g., lysosomal DNase II), which derives from the cells that have phagocytized the apoptotic remnants or destroy the DNA that is released into the extracellular compartment.

Under physiological conditions, the intracellular nucleases involved in apoptosis are confined to the cell. However, if cells lyse during blood collection, storage, or handling, they will be released into the specimen (e.g., serum or plasma) and could contribute to the ex vivo DNA-degrading activity of the sample. While the appearance of genomic DNA in cirDNA isolated from plasma, concomitant with an unexpectedly high measurement of DNA concentration, can be indicative of cell lysis and contamination with cellular components, absence of genomic DNA does not necessarily exclude that cytoplasmic cell contents haven't been released.

The nucleus, supported by the nuclear lamina, is relatively robust and lysis of the plasma membrane is likely to precede lysis of the nucleus.[80] Isolated cell nuclei are pelleted by relatively low centrifugation speeds (e.g., 800 × g),[81] such as are typically used to separate plasma from cellular blood components. Hence, nuclei from partially lysed cells, if present, will be separated from plasma during blood centrifugation along with red blood cells and leukocytes, and an absence of genomic DNA in the sample does not necessarily indicate that the plasma hasn't been contaminated with cytoplasmic contents. The same considerations apply to serum, which is well known to have a higher cirDNA concentration than plasma, and this increased concentration has been attributed to cell lysis during the coagulation.[79] Hence, intracellular DNAses involved in apoptosis are described in the following, and their activity profile and characteristics are summarized in Table 2.

Caspase-Activated DNase

CAD, also called DFF40, is characterized by neutral pH optimum, Mg^{2+} requirement, and formation of DNA reaction products with a hydroxyl group at the 3'-end and a phosphate group at the 5'-end. It is specific for double-stranded DNA not for single stranded DNA or RNA and exhibits an extraordinary preference for cleaving the internucleosomal linker regions in chromatin (the enzyme is unable to cut DNA bound to the histone octamer).[82] The enzyme cuts both DNA strands and generates blunt ends or ends with 1-base 5'-overhangs.[83] Consequently, its action on chromatin results in the classical DNA ladders observed upon apoptotic cell death (~180 pb periodicity).[84] CAD is found in the cell nuclei and cytoplasm heterodimerized with its inhibitor, which is released upon apoptotic activation.[85]

Endonuclease G

Endonuclease G is a mitochondrial nuclease that translocates to the nucleus during apoptosis.[86] The enzyme is characterized by neutral pH optimum, Mg^{2+} or Mn^{2+} ion requirement, and formation of DNA reaction products with a hydroxyl group at the 3′-end and a phosphate group at the 5′-end. Endonuclease G "prefers" single-stranded DNA or RNA over double-stranded DNA.[87] Endonuclease G chromatin cleavage often results in single-stranded nicks between nucleosomes in the DNA linkers (~190 bases periodicity) and within the nucleosome core (~10 base periodicity).[88] These cleavage patterns are similar to those of DNase I digestion products.[89] However, unlike DNase I, Endonuclease G preferentially attacks single-stranded regions, allowing for targeting by single-stranded nicks for adjacent strand cleavage to generate double-stranded nucleosomal length fragments.[88] DNase I and exonuclease III stimulate its ability to generate dsDNA cleavage products at physiological ionic strength in vitro.[88]

DNAse γ

DNase γ is characterized by neutral pH optimum, Ca^{2+} and Mg^{2+} requirement, and formation of single-stranded DNA breaks with a hydroxyl group at the 3′-end and a phosphate group at the 5′-end. The enzyme is stored in the nuclear envelope lumen and released into the nucleus in the late apoptotic phase and accelerates DNA fragmentation. Thus, DNA fragmentation is initiated by CAD/DFF40 and DNase γ completes the digestion of the genomic DNA in dying cells as apoptosis' final caretaker.[90] The enzyme action on naked DNA generates the typical DNA ladder as seen in apoptosis but only at low ionic strength buffer conditions. However, in the presence of histone H1, the DNase γ coactivator, naked DNA, and chromatin are effectively cleaved at physiological ionic strength.[91]

Leukocyte Elastase Inhibitor-Derived DNAse II (L-DNase II)

Leukocyte Elastase Inhibitor (LEI)-derived DNase II (L-DNase II) is characterized by acidic pH optimum, bivalent ions independency, and formation DNA breaks with a hydroxyl group at the 5′-end and a phosphate group at the 3′-end.[87] The enzyme induces the cleavage of DNA into an oligonucleosomal ladder in vitro.[92] Curiously, L-DNAse II originates from the LEI, a member of the serine protease inhibitors superfamily. The acidic treatment or action of some proteases (e.g., elastase, cathepsin D, and other proteases activated during apoptosis) over LEI changes its enzymatic activity; the antiprotease activity is lost and the endonuclease activity is gained. The modification also unveils a nuclear localization signal. Hence, L-DNAse II enters into the nucleus, cleaves the DNA, and finally leads to apoptosis.[93] This is a caspase-independent pathway and an interesting example in which an anti-apoptotic protein acquires pro-apoptotic function.[87]

Other Apoptosis DNases

There are several other less characterized apoptosis DNases — for review see.[86,87]

Clinical Correlates of Blood DNAse I Activity

Serum DNase I activity has been measured in several diseases/conditions (Table 3). If compared to the levels found in healthy

Table 3. Diseases or Conditions with High/Low Serum DNase I Activity Compared to Controls

High serum DNase I activity	Low serum DNase I activity
Oral cancer[94]	Malignant lymphomas[95]
Breast cancer[96]	Stomach and colon cancer[11]
Transient myocardial ischaemia[97,98]	Pancreatic cancer and pancreatitis[99]
Acute myocardial infarction[100]	Overnight fast[101]
Antineutrophil cytoplasmic antibody-associated vasculitis[102]	Surgical trauma[101]
Type 2 diabetes[103]	Systemic lupus erythematosus[104,105]
Exercise[106]	Prostate tumors[10]

individuals, blood DNA-degrading activity can be classified into two categories: high serum DNase activity compared to controls or low serum DNase activity compared to controls (see below). Although the focus of intensive research, the diagnostic utility of serum DNAse activity has not been translated to clinical practice yet. Differences in the methods used, low-level of enzymatic activity, and large inter-individual variations are some of the factors that contribute to this scenario.[58]

Assays to Monitor the DNase Activity

Fluorometric, electrochemical, and immunological assays have been developed to monitor the DNase activity in clinical samples; further details can be found in the review by Sato and Takenaka.[107] The fluorometric assays can be divided into three classes (Fig. 2).

Assay Based on Decrease in Fluorescence of Noncovalent DNA Dyes

These assays rely on the fact that noncovalent DNA dyes (e.g., Pico Green, SYBR Green, or ethidium bromide) fluoresce when

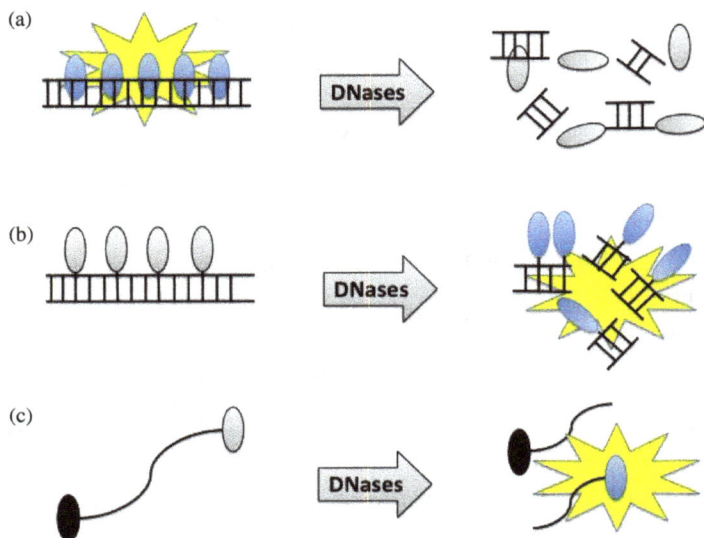

Fig. 2:   The principles of fluorometric assays to monitor the DNAse activity in clinical samples: (a) assays based on decrease in fluorescence of DNA intercalating dyes; (b) assays based on increase in fluorescence of attenuated DNA dyes; (c) assays based on cleavage of dual-labeled probes. Attenuated dyes (grey ellipses), deattenuated dyes (blue ellipses), and quencher (black ellipse).

bound to double-stranded DNA molecules. The degradation of the double-stranded DNA molecules by DNases decreases the fluorescence, which is proportional to the enzyme activity (Fig. 2a).[108] These assays can be performed in solution or in a matrix (e.g., agarose gels — the single radial enzyme-diffusion assay).[48,109]

Assays Based on Increase in Fluorescence Self-attenuated Covalent DNA Dyes

These assays use DNA molecules covalently conjugated to a fluorescent dye. The proximity with the DNA attenuates its fluorescence. With DNA cleavage by Dnases, the fluorescence increases proportionally to the enzyme activity (Fig. 2b).[110]

Assays Based on Fluorescence Deattenuation of Dual-labeled Probes (e.g., qPCR Hydrolysis Probes)

These assays use single-stranded oligonucleotides labeled with a fluorophore and a quencher. The oligo cleavage by DNAses physically separates both labels, and the fluorescence increase reports the enzyme activity (Fig. 2c).[111,112]

DNAse Activity and the Initial Circulation Cell-Free DNA Concentration in Plasmas and Serum

Blood nucleases degrade cirDNA ex vivo and are a preanalytical source of variation that decreases the sensitivity of molecular assays. For many years, their impact on cirDNA was neglected.[113] Our group conceived independently an assay based on a qPCR hydrolysis probe degradation to monitor the DNase activity in clinical samples. However, previous similar protocols were identified after a literature search. By using this method, we measured blood DNase activity in the major cell-free specimens: plasma-EDTA, plasma-heparin, plasma-citrate 3.2%, and serum.[113,114]

Endogenous DNase Activity Assay

Endogenous DNase activity assay consisted of the admixture of the crude sample with a qPCR hydrolysis probe in a qPCR master mix. The reactions were then incubated isothermally at 37°C for 24 hr on a qPCR system. The fluorescence is measured every 30 min. The qPCR master mix contains ROX (passive reference dye) and probe labeled with FAM (active dye). When the hydrolysis probe is intact, the quencher is close to FAM and its fluorescence is mitigated. The FAM fluorescence increases upon hydrolysis probe cleavage by DNase activity of the sample. The unit of the

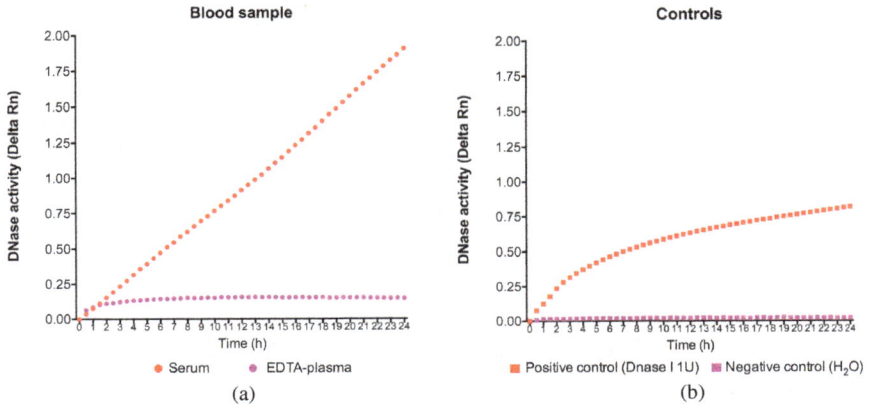

Fig. 3: qPCR hydrolysis probe kinetics observed in the endogenous DNase activity assay for (a) plasma-EDTA (magenta circles) and serum (red circles) and (b) 1U of DNase I (red squares) and H_2O (magenta squares).

reaction is the deltaRn, which is the ratio of fluorescence values between active and passive dyes in each measurement subtracted by the ratio of the first measurement. A typical graphical representation of the endogenous DNase activity assay in paired plasma-EDTA and serum samples is shown in Fig. 3 (a plot of deltaRn versus time).[113]

Plasma-EDTA

Endogenous DNase activity is highly inhibited in plasma-EDTA (Fig. 2a). It makes this matrix the specimen of choice to avoid the DNases' ex vivo impact on cirDNA. Indeed, EDTA works as an indirect inhibitor. This anticoagulant chelates divalent ions (Ca^{2+}, Mg^{2+} and Mn^{2+}), which are essential for the activity of many DNAses, especially DNAse I (the major DNase found in blood) providing higher stability to the analyte.[113]

Although the inhibition is high, it is not complete. A residual DNase activity is observed in plasma-EDTA and it could be

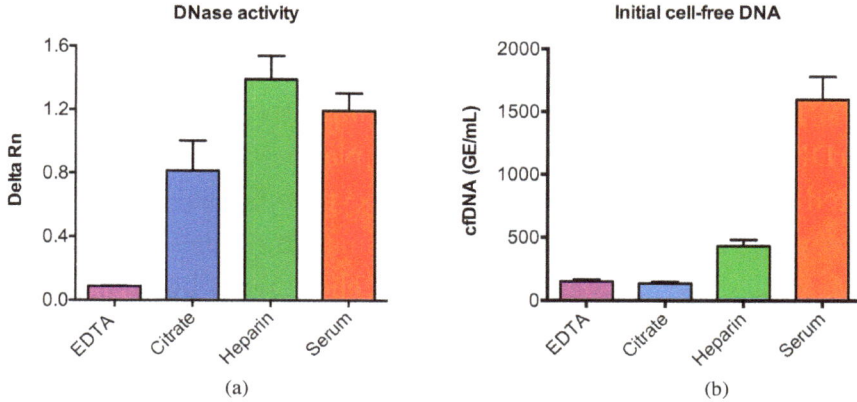

Fig. 4: DNase activity (a) and initial cirDNA (b) of the main plasma tube types and serum.

attributed to the following: (a) the concentration of EDTA in regular tubes is not enough for full inhibition[113] and (b) the small concentration of DNAse II found in blood, an enzyme that is independent of bivalent ions (Fig. 4a).

Another advantage of the plasma-EDTA is that the original admixture of DNA sequences found in the bloodstream tends to be preserved in this specimen, because of the low contamination with leukocyte genomic DNA in promptly processed blood samples.[115] Such contamination could decrease the cirDNA assay sensitivity for rare DNA sequences. Consequently, plasma-EDTA better represents the physiological status of the cirDNA in vivo[114] (Fig. 4b).

Plasma-Citrate 3.2%

Similar to EDTA, sodium citrate is an anticoagulant that chelates bivalent ions.[116,117] However, blood DNase activity of this specimen is only partially inhibited in the endogenous DNase activity assay.[114] This may be due to the sodium citrate concentration in the collection tube being lower than the optimum for full enzymatic inhibition (Fig. 4a).

Moreover, just after the blood draw, the initial amount of cirDNA in this specimen is similar to plasma-EDTA. The above-cited lower contamination with leukocyte genomic DNA is also observed. These results make the plasma-citrate the best alternative to plasma-EDTA and suggest that chelating of bivalent ions is a mechanism to both inhibit blood DNAses and avoid the introduction of unnecessary DNA sequences to the specimen[114] (Fig. 4b).

Plasma-Heparin

Among the tested specimens, plasma-heparin showed the highest DNase activity in the endogenous DNase activity assay (Fig. 4a). It is 17-fold higher compared to plasma-EDTA.[114] The mechanism by which heparin prevents blood coagulation is not based on divalent cation chelation. The anticoagulant action of heparin lies in its ability to bind to and enhance the inhibitory activity of the plasma protein antithrombin against several serine proteases of the coagulation system, most importantly factors IIa (thrombin), Xa and IXa.[118] Because DNase activity is a temperature-triggered mechanism,[113] strictly low-temperature condition control should be applied to heparin samples to neutralize the DNases' ex vivo impact on cirDNA (it can be more flexible for plasma-EDTA). On the other hand, the initial amount of cirDNA in this specimen is slightly higher compared to the paired plasma-EDTA and plasma-citrate (Fig. 4b). It suggests a small contamination with leukocyte's genomic DNA after the blood draw, which could be explained by direct effect of heparin over these cells.[119] Again, ex vivo introduction of unnecessary nucleic acids could decrease the cirDNA assay sensitivity for rare DNA sequences. Taken together, these observations indicate that plasma-heparin should be avoided in cirDNA studies and analyses.

Serum

Serum has second highest DNase activity among the tested specimens, which is 15-fold higher than plasma-EDTA (Fig. 4a). To neutralize the DNases' ex vivo impact on cirDNA, the strictly low-temperature condition control should also be applied to serum samples.[113] Moreover, due to leukocyte lysis during coagulation, a phenomenon not fully understood yet, serum is highly contaminated with genomic DNA (Fig. 4b).[114] Thus, as with heparin, serum's cell-free DNA admixture doesn't reflect the in vivo condition, and consequently should be avoided in cirDNA studies and analyses. Conversely, serum is an acceptable alternative to whole blood for patient genomic DNA analysis.[120]

Nonanticoagulated Plasma

The nonanticoagulated plasma is obtained by blood draw in a plain tube followed by immediate centrifugation. Probably, this is the specimen that best represents the in vivo physiological status of blood DNases and cell-free DNA, but is difficult to obtain and handle. We observed similar DNA-degrading activity in nonanticoagulated plasma as in paired serum, although they were different between individuals,[113] suggesting that lysis of leukocytes and release of cellular contents do not alter the nuclease profile of serum compared to nonanticoagulated plasma. However, further experiments are required to reach the final conclusion on this question (Fig. 4).

Influence of Temperature

Blood DNase activity is a temperature-dependent mechanism[113] and temperature is an important preanalytical factor for specimens that lack additives with bivalent ion chelation capacity (e.g., serum and plasma-heparin).[114] In serum, no difference is observed in the cirDNA yield after incubation at –20°C and 4°C for 24 hr, otherwise, a decrease occurs at room temperature and 37°C. Because EDTA indirectly inhibits blood DNases, the cirDNA is protected from degradation in plasma-EDTA at 37°C (at least for 24 hr). Despite the EDTA inhibition, the small but still detectable nuclease activity leads to a significant reduction of the cirDNA yield after 48 hr at 37°C.[113]

EDTA Concentration

The addition of a 10-fold serial dilution of EDTA to nonanticoagulated plasma (and also to serum) resulted in a stepwise reduction of the blood DNase activity, evidencing that EDTA indirectly inhibits blood's DNases.[113] However, the EDTA concentration in regular EDTA tubes ranges from 1.5 to 2.0 mg per mL of blood,[121] corresponding to approximately 5×10^{-3} M. We observed a significant but not complete inhibition of the DNase activity at this concentration. These results suggest that the cirDNA assays would benefit from a 10-fold increase of EDTA concentration in the collection tube since no or negligible DNAse activity was observed at 5×10^{-2} M (Fig. 4).[113]

Other Known Factors

Considering the remnant blood DNase activity ex vivo in regular EDTA tubes, cirDNA analysis could benefit from a 10-fold increase of EDTA concentration in the collection tubes (Fig. 5).

Nonanticoagulated plasma

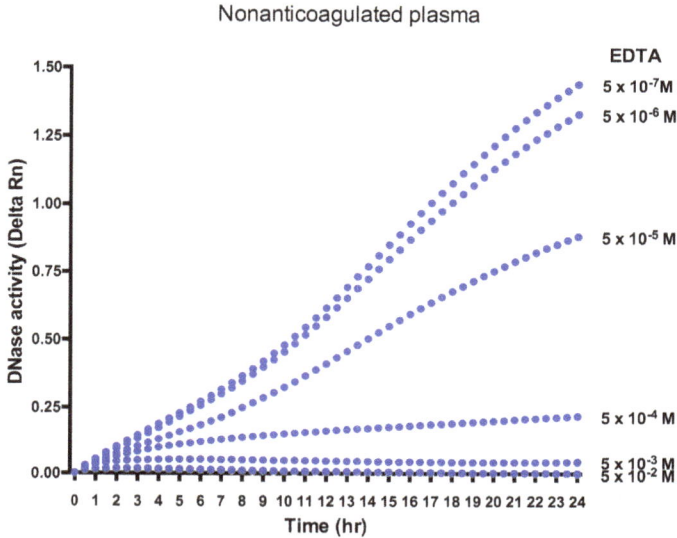

Fig. 5: A serial dilution of EDTA was added to nonanticoagulated plasma before the endogenous DNase activity assay in order to investigate the EDTA-mediated inhibition of hydrolysis probe degradation. A stepwise inhibition of the hydrolysis probe degradation was observed, consistent with EDTA indirectly inhibiting the sample's DNase activity.

Tube manufacturers should consider producing such a tube, specifically for the liquid biopsy field. Moreover, in the endogenous DNase activity assay, the positive control showed hydrolysis probe degradation kinetics that was not as continuous as the serum samples. We cannot distinguish if this effect is secondary to a higher DNase amount in the serum together with the presence of inhibitors, or secondary to the complex composition of DNA-degrading enzymes in serum (Fig. 3).[113]

Approaches to Minimizing Preanalytical Artifacts in cirDNA Analysis

The aim of cirDNA assays and studies is frequently the detection of rare tumoral or fetal sequences in a huge background of wild-type or maternal DNA, respectively. With the blood drawn, the supply of these rare DNA sequences terminates and they become exposed to the blood DNA-degrading activity, which could decrease the assay sensitivity. Moreover, the ex vivo introduction of nucleic acids from leukocytes further dilutes the signal and should also be avoided. In summary, to minimize these preanalytical effects over circulation cell-free DNA the following recommendations should be considered:

(1) Use a collection tube with a DNase inhibitor (e.g., EDTA) to minimize the enzyme action during blood processing, transportation, and storage.
(2) Avoid coagulation and leukocyte lysis.
(3) Process the blood into its cell-free subproducts and/or physically separate the cellular content as soon as possible avoiding unwanted DNA contamination (e.g., centrifugation and aliquoting or blood draw in tubes with gel barrier).
(4) Transport the sample at refrigerator temperature (2°C to 8°C) or less, as DNAse activity is a temperature-triggered enzymatic activity.
(5) Plan to extract the DNA and detect the rare DNA as soon as possible, as it is difficult to neutralize all DNAse activity.
6) If necessary, store the crude sample at freezer temperature (−12°C to −20°C) or less.

Limitations of Current Knowledge

The limitations of the current knowledge are:

a) Relative contribution of apoptosis, necrosis, netosis, and other mechanisms to the cirDNA pool under pathological conditions.

b) Complete understanding of the cirDNA clearance from circulation, including the relative contribution of DNases, intake by cells, and liver and kidney metabolism.

c) The diagnostic utility and clinical application of blood DNAse activity measurement.

d) Why DNase activity of the serum has a different kinetics when compared to the DNase I positive control in endogenous DNase activity assay.

e) How to inhibit both bivalent metal ion dependent and independent DNases ex vivo in the collection tube for cirDNA analysis.

f) Exact mechanism by which the blood clot formation introduces genomic DNA into serum.

References

1. Jung K, Fleischhacker M, Rabien A. (2010) Cell-free DNA in the blood as a solid tumor biomarker — a critical appraisal of the literature. *Clin Chim Acta* **411**: 1611–1624.

2. Chiou HC, Tangco MV, Levine SM, *et al*. (1994) Enhanced resistance to nuclease degradation of nucleic acids complexed to asialoglycoprotein-polylysine carriers. *Nucleic Acids Res* **22**: 5439–5446.

3. Cox RA, Gokcen M. (1976) Comparison of serum DNA, native DNA-binding and deoxyribonuclease levels in ten animal species and man. *Life Sci* **19**: 1609–1614.

4. Wickstrom E. (1986) Oligodeoxynucleotide stability in subcellular extracts and culture media. *J Biochem Biophys Methods* **13**: 97–102.

5. Agrawal S, Temsamani J, Galbraith W, Tang J. (1995) Pharmacokinetics of antisense oligonucleotides. *Clin Pharmacokinet* **28**: 7–16.

6. Geary RS, Norris D, Yu R, Bennett CF. (2015) Pharmacokinetics, biodistribution and cell uptake of antisense oligonucleotides. *Adv Drug Delivery Rev* **87**: 46–51.

7. Baranovskii AG, Buneva VN, Nevinsky GA. (2004) Human deoxyribonucleases. *Biochem Biokhimiia* **69**: 587–601.

8. Peters DL, Pretorius PJ. (2011) Origin, translocation and destination of
extracellular occurring DNA — a new paradigm in genetic behaviour.
Clin Chim Acta **412**: 806–811.

9. van der Vaart M, Pretorius PJ. (2007) The origin of circulating free DNA.
Clin Chem **53**: 2215.

10. Cherepanova AV, Tamkovich SN, Bryzgunova OE, *et al.* (2008) Deoxyribonuclease activity and circulating DNA concentration in blood plasma of
patients with prostate tumors. *Ann N Y Acad Sci* **1137**: 218–221.

11. Tamkovich SN, Cherepanova AV, Kolesnikova EV, *et al.* (2006) Circulating DNA and DNase activity in human blood. *Ann N Y Acad Sci* **1075**:
191–196.

12. Napirei M, Karsunky H, Zevnik B, *et al.* (2000) Features of systemic lupus
erythematosus in Dnase1-deficient mice. *Nat Genet* **25**: 177–181.

13. Yasutomo K, Horiuchi T, Kagami S, *et al.* (2001) Mutation of DNASE1 in
people with systemic lupus erythematosus. *Nat Genet* **28**: 313–314.

14. Martinez Valle F, Balada E, Ordi-Ros J, Vilardell-Tarres M. (2008) DNase
1 and systemic lupus erythematosus. *Autoimmun Rev* **7**: 359–363.

15. Gaipl US, Beyer TD, Heyder P, *et al.* (2004) Cooperation between C1q
and DNase I in the clearance of necrotic cell-derived chromatin. *Arthritis
Rheum* **50**: 640–649.

16. Stephan F, Marsman G, Bakker LM, *et al.* (2014) Cooperation of factor
VII-activating protease and serum DNase I in the release of nucleosomes
from necrotic cells. *Arthritis Rheum* **66**: 686–693.

17. Liang YY, Rainprecht D, Eichmair E, *et al.* (2015) Serum-dependent processing of late apoptotic cells and their immunogenicity. *Apoptosis Int J
Program Cell Death* **20**: 1444–1456.

18. Yu SC, Lee SW, Jiang P, *et al.* (2013) High-resolution profiling of fetal
DNA clearance from maternal plasma by massively parallel sequencing.
Clin Chem **59**: 1228–1237.

19. Lo YM, Zhang J, Leung TN, *et al.* (1999) Rapid clearance of fetal DNA
from maternal plasma. *Am J Hum Genet* **64**: 218–224.

20. Botezatu I, Serdyuk O, Potapova G, *et al.* (2000) Genetic analysis of DNA
excreted in urine: a new approach for detecting specific genomic DNA
sequences from cells dying in an organism. *Clin Chem* **46**: 1078–1084.

21. Diehl F, Schmidt K, Choti MA, *et al.* (2008) Circulating mutant DNA to assess tumor dynamics. *Nat Med* **14**: 985–990.

22. Snyder MW, Kircher M, Hill AJ, *et al.* (2016) Cell-free DNA comprises an *in vivo* nucleosome footprint that informs its tissues-of-origin. *Cell* **164**: 57–68.

23. Fleischhacker M, Schmidt B. (2007) Circulating nucleic acids (CNAs) and cancer — a survey. *Biochimica et Biophysica Acta* **1775**: 181–232.

24. Giacona MB, Ruben GC, Iczkowski KA, *et al.* (1998) Cell-free DNA in human blood plasma: length measurements in patients with pancreatic cancer and healthy controls. *Pancreas* **17**: 89–97.

25. Wyllie AH, Morris RG, Smith AL, Dunlop D. (1984) Chromatin cleavage in apoptosis: association with condensed chromatin morphology and dependence on macromolecular synthesis. *J Pathol* **142**: 67–77.

26. Opferman JT. (2007) Life and death during hematopoietic differentiation. *Curr Opin Immunol* **19**: 497–502.

27. Stroun M, Lyautey J, Lederrey C, *et al.* (2001) About the possible origin and mechanism of circulating DNA apoptosis and active DNA release. *Clin Chim Acta* **313**: 139–142.

28. Jahr S, Hentze H, Englisch S, *et al.* (2001) DNA fragments in the blood plasma of cancer patients: quantitations and evidence for their origin from apoptotic and necrotic cells. *Cancer Res* **61**: 1659–1665.

29. Yipp BG, Kubes P. (2013) NETosis: how vital is it? *Blood* **122**: 2784–2794.

30. Manda A, Pruchniak MP, Arazna M, Demkow UA. (2014) Neutrophil extracellular traps in physiology and pathology. *Cent Eur J Immunol* **39**: 116–121.

31. Jiang P, Lo YM. (2016) The long and short of circulating cell-free DNA and the ins and outs of molecular diagnostics. *Trends Genet* **32**(6): 360–371.

32. Chandrananda D, Thorne NP, Bahlo M. (2015) High-resolution characterization of sequence signatures due to non-random cleavage of cell-free DNA. *BMC Med Genom* **8**: 29.

33. Lo YM, Chan KC, Sun H, *et al.* (2010) Maternal plasma DNA sequencing reveals the genome-wide genetic and mutational profile of the fetus. *Sci Transl Med* **2**: 61ra91.

34. Cheng SH, Jiang P, Sun K, *et al.* (2015) Noninvasive prenatal testing by nanopore sequencing of maternal plasma DNA: feasibility assessment. *Clin Chem* **61**: 1305–1306.

35. Solovyan VT, Bezvenyuk ZA, Salminen A, *et al.* (2002) The role of topoisomerase II in the excision of DNA loop domains during apoptosis. *J Biol Chem* **277**: 21458–21467.

36. Susin SA, Lorenzo HK, Zamzami N, *et al.* (1999) Molecular characterization of mitochondrial apoptosis-inducing factor. *Nature* **397**: 441–446.

37. Widlak P. (2000) The DFF40/CAD endonuclease and its role in apoptosis. *Acta Biochim Pol* **47**: 1037–1044.

38. Liu X, Zou H, Slaughter C, Wang X. (1997) DFF, a heterodimeric protein that functions downstream of caspase-3 to trigger DNA fragmentation during apoptosis. *Cell* **89**: 175–184.

39. Enari M, Sakahira H, Yokoyama H, *et al.* (1998) A caspase-activated DNase that degrades DNA during apoptosis, and its inhibitor ICAD. *Nature* **391**: 43–50.

40. Li LY, Luo X, Wang X. (2001) Endonuclease G is an apoptotic DNase when released from mitochondria. *Nature* **412**: 95–99.

41. Oliveri M, Daga A, Cantoni C, *et al.* (2001) DNase I mediates internucleosomal DNA degradation in human cells undergoing drug-induced apoptosis. *Eur J Immunol* **31**: 743–751.

42. Elmore S. (2007) Apoptosis: a review of programmed cell death. *Toxicol Pathol* **35**: 495–516.

43. Kawane K, Nagata S. (2008) Nucleases in programmed cell death. *Methods Enzymol* **442**: 271–287.

44. Bischoff FZ, Lewis DE, Simpson JL. (2005) Cell-free fetal DNA in maternal blood: kinetics, source and structure. *Hum Reprod Update* **11**: 59–67.

45. Hariton-Gazal E, Rosenbluh J, Graessmann A, *et al.* (2003) Direct translocation of histone molecules across cell membranes. *J Cell Sci* **116**: 4577–4586.

46. Luger K. (2003) Structure and dynamic behavior of nucleosomes. *Curr Opin Genet Dev* **13**: 127–135.

47. Westheimer FH. (1987) Why nature chose phosphates. *Science* **235**: 1173–1178.

48. Nadano D, Yasuda T, Kishi K. (1993) Measurement of deoxyribonuclease I activity in human tissues and body fluids by a single radial enzyme-diffusion method. *Clin Chem* **39**: 448–452.

49. Gueroult M, Picot D, Abi-Ghanem J, *et al.* (2010) How cations can assist DNase I in DNA binding and hydrolysis. *PLoS Comput Biol* **6**: e1001000.

50. Moore S. (1981) Pancreatic DNase. In: PD Boyer (eds), *The Enzymes*, Academic Press, New York, pp. 281–296.

51. Drew HR. (1984) Structural specificities of five commonly used DNA nucleases. *J Mol Biol* **176**: 535–557.

52. Weston SA, Lahm A, Suck D. (1992) X-ray structure of the DNase I-d(G-GTATACC)2 complex at 2.3 A resolution. *J Mol Biol* **226**: 1237–1256.

53. Lahm A, Suck D. (1991) DNase I-induced DNA conformation. 2 A structure of a DNase I-octamer complex. *J Mol Biol* **222**: 645–667.

54. Riley DE. (1980) Deoxyribonuclease I generates single-stranded gaps in chromatin deoxyribonucleic acid. *Biochemistry* **19**: 2977–2992.

55. Noll M. (1974) Internal structure of the chromatin subunit. *Nucleic Acids Res* **1**: 1573–1578.

56. Cousins DJ, Islam SA, Sanderson MR, *et al.* (2004) Redefinition of the cleavage sites of DNase I on the nucleosome core particle. *J Mol Biol* **335**: 1199–1211.

57. Lazarus RA, Wagener JA. (2013) *Recombinant Human Deoxyribonuclease I. Pharmaceutical Biotechnology*. Springer, New York, pp. 321–336.

58. Cherepanova A, Tamkovich S, Pyshnyi D, *et al.* (2007) Immunochemical assay for deoxyribonuclease activity in body fluids. *J Immunol Methods* **325**: 96–103.

59. Sierakowska H, Shugar D. (1977) Mammalian nucleolytic enzymes. *Prog Nucl Acid Res Mol Biol* **20**: 59–130.

60. Evans CJ, Aguilera RJ. (2003) DNase II: genes, enzymes and function. *Gene* **322**: 1–15.

61. Murai K, Yamanaka M, Akagi K, Anai M. (1980) Purification and properties of deoxyribonuclease II from human urine. *J Biochem* **87**: 1097–1103.

62. Baker KP, Baron WF, Henzel WJ, Spencer SA. (1998) Molecular cloning and characterization of human and murine DNase II. *Gene* **215**: 281–289.

63. Gross SC, Watabe M, Goodarzi G, *et al.* (1990) Organ-specific distribution of isozymes of 5´-nucleotide phosphodiesterase in mouse. *Comp Biochem Physiol B Comp Biochem* **95**: 821–824.

64. Luthje J, Ogilvie A. (1987) 5′-Nucleotide phosphodiesterase isoenzymes in human serum: quantitative measurement and some biochemical properties. *Clin Chim Acta* **164**: 275–284.

65. Eder PS, DeVine RJ, Dagle JM, Walder JA. (1991) Substrate specificity and kinetics of degradation of antisense oligonucleotides by a 3′ exonuclease in plasma. *Antisense Res Dev* **1**: 141–151.

66. Ito K, Yamamoto T, Minamiura N. (1987) Phosphodiesterase I in human urine: purification and characterization of the enzyme. *J Biochem* **102**: 359–367.

67. Goding JW, Terkeltaub R, Maurice M, *et al.* (1998) Ecto-phosphodiesterase/pyrophosphatase of lymphocytes and non-lymphoid cells: structure and function of the PC-1 family. *Immunol Rev* **161**: 11–26.

68. Hynie I, Meuffels M, Poznanski WJ. (1975) Determination of phosphodiesterase I activity in human blood serum. *Clin Chem* **21**: 1383–1387.

69. Frittitta L, Camastra S, Baratta R, *et al.* (1999) A soluble PC-1 circulates in human plasma: relationship with insulin resistance and associated abnormalities. *J Clin Endocrinol Metabol* **84**: 3620–3625.

70. Belli SI, Goding JW. (1994) Biochemical characterization of human PC-1, an enzyme possessing alkaline phosphodiesterase I and nucleotide pyrophosphatase activities. *Eur J Biochem / FEBS* **226**: 433–443.

71. Shuster AM, Gololobov GV, Kvashuk OA, *et al.* (1992) DNA hydrolyzing autoantibodies. *Science* **256**: 665–667.

72. Baranovskii AG, Ershova NA, Buneva VN, *et al.* (2001) Catalytic heterogeneity of polyclonal DNA-hydrolyzing antibodies from the sera of patients with multiple sclerosis. *Immunol Lett* **76**: 163–167.

73. Cherepanova AV, Tamkovich SN, Vlasov VV, Laktionov PP. (2007) Blood deoxyribonuclease activity in health and diseases. *Biomeditsinskaia khimiia* **53**: 488–496.

74. Babina SE, Kanyshkova TG, Buneva VN, Nevinsky GA. (2004) Lactoferrin is the major deoxyribonuclease of human milk. *Biochem Biokhimiia* **69**: 1006–1015.

75. Masson PL, Heremans JF, Dive CH. (1966) An iron-binding protein common to many external secretions. *Clin Chim Acta* **14**: 5.

76. Masson PL, Heremans JF, Schonne E. (1969) Lactoferrin, an iron-binding protein in neutrophilic leukocytes. *J Exper Med* **130**: 643–658.

77. Bennett RM, Kokocinski T. (1979) Lactoferrin turnover in man. *Clin Sci* **57**: 453–460.

78. Barthe C, Galabert C, Guy-Crotte O, Figarella C. (1989) Plasma and serum lactoferrin levels in cystic fibrosis. Relationship with the presence of cystic fibrosis protein. *Clin Chim Acta* **181**: 183–188.

79. Lee TH, Montalvo L, Chrebtow V, Busch MP. (2001) Quantitation of genomic DNA in plasma and serum samples: higher concentrations of genomic DNA found in serum than in plasma. *Transfusion* **41**: 276–282.

80. Grandinetti G, Smith AE, Reineke TM. (2012) Membrane and nuclear permeabilization by polymeric pDNA vehicles: efficient method for gene delivery or mechanism of cytotoxicity? *Mol Pharm* **9**: 523–538.

81. Valenzuela SM, Martin DK, Por SB, *et al.* (1997) Molecular cloning and expression of a chloride ion channel of cell nuclei. *J Biol Chem* **272**: 12575–12582.

82. Widlak P, Garrard WT. (2006) Unique features of the apoptotic endonuclease DFF40/CAD relative to micrococcal nuclease as a structural probe for chromatin. *Biochem Cell Biol* **84**: 405–410.

83. Widlak P, Li P, Wang X, Garrard WT. (2000) Cleavage preferences of the apoptotic endonuclease DFF40 (caspase-activated DNase or nuclease) on naked DNA and chromatin substrates. *J Biol Chem* **275**: 8226–8232.

84. Allan J, Fraser RM, Owen-Hughes T, Keszenman-Pereyra D. (2012) Micrococcal nuclease does not substantially bias nucleosome mapping. *J Mol Biol* **417**: 152–164.

85. Woo EJ, Kim YG, Kim MS, *et al.* (2004) Structural mechanism for inactivation and activation of CAD/DFF40 in the apoptotic pathway. *Mol Cell* **14**: 531–539.

86. Counis MF, Torriglia A. (2006) Acid DNases and their interest among apoptotic endonucleases. *Biochimie* **88**: 1851–1858.

87. Samejima K, Earnshaw WC. (2005) Trashing the genome: the role of nucleases during apoptosis. *Nat Rev Mol Cell Biol* **6**: 677–688.

88. Widlak P, Li LY, Wang X, Garrard WT. (2001) Action of recombinant human apoptotic endonuclease G on naked DNA and chromatin substrates: cooperation with exonuclease and DNase I. *J Biol Chem* **276**: 48404–48409.

89. Lutter LC. (1979) Precise location of DNase I cutting sites in the nucleosome core determined by high resolution gel electrophoresis. *Nucleic Acids Res* **6**: 41–56.

90. Mizuta R, Mizuta M, Araki S, *et al.* (2009) DNase gamma-dependent and -independent apoptotic DNA fragmentations in Ramos Burkitt's lymphoma cell line. *Biomed Res* **30**: 165–170.

91. Mizuta R, Mizuta M, Araki S, *et al.* (2006) Action of apoptotic endonuclease DNase gamma on naked DNA and chromatin substrates. *Biochem Biophy Res Commun* **345**: 560–567.

92. Torriglia A, Perani P, Brossas JY, *et al.* (1998) L-DNase II, a molecule that links proteases and endonucleases in apoptosis, derives from the ubiquitous serpin leukocyte elastase inhibitor. *Mol Cell Biol* **18**: 3612–3619.

93. Torriglia A, Martin E, Jaadane I. (2017) The hidden side of SERPINB1/ Leukocyte Elastase Inhibitor. *Semin Cell Develop Biol* **62**: 178–186.

94. Scully C, Spandidos DA, Ward Booth P, *et al.* (1981) Serum alkaline deoxyribonuclease in oral cancer and premalignant lesions. *Biomedicine / [publiee pour l'AAICIG]* **35**: 179–180.

95. Economidou-Karaoglou A, Lans M, Taper HS, *et al.* (1988) Variations in serum alkaline DNase activity. A new means for therapeutic monitoring of malignant lymphomas. *Cancer* **61**: 1838–1843.

96. Spandidos DA, Ramandanis G, Garas J, Kottaridis SD. (1980) Serum deoxyribonucleases in patients with breast cancer. *Eur J Cancer* **16**: 1615–1619.

97. Arakawa K, Kawai Y, Kumamoto T, *et al.* (2005) Serum deoxyribonuclease I activity can be used as a sensitive marker for detection of transient myocardial ischaemia induced by percutaneous coronary intervention. *Eur Heart J* **26**: 2375–2380.

98. Morikawa N, Kawai Y, Arakawa K, *et al.* (2007) Serum deoxyribonuclease I activity can be used as a novel marker of transient myocardial ischaemia: results in vasospastic angina pectoris induced by provocation test. *Eur Heart J* **28**: 2992–2997.

99. Funakoshi A, Wakasugi H, Ibayashi H. (1979) Clinical investigation of serum deoxyribonuclease: II. Clinical studies of serum deoxyribonuclease activity in pancreatic disease. *Gastroenterol Jpn* **14**: 436–440.

100. Kuribara J, Tada H, Kawai Y, *et al*. (2009) Levels of serum deoxyribonuclease I activity on admission in patients with acute myocardial infarction can be useful in predicting left ventricular enlargement due to remodeling. *J Cardiol* **53**: 196–203.

101. Lundqvist EH, Sjovall K, Eneroth PH. (1992) Influences of diet and surgical trauma on serum alkaline DNase activity levels. *Clin Chim Acta* **205**: 43–49.

102. Wang H, Sha LL, Ma TT, *et al*. (2016) Circulating level of neutrophil extracellular traps is not a useful biomarker for assessing disease activity in antineutrophil cytoplasmic antibody-associated vasculitis. *PloS One* **11**: e0148197.

103. Zhu B, Gong Y, Chen P, *et al*. (2014) Increased DNase I activity in diabetes might be associated with injury of pancreas. *Mol Cell Biochem* **393**: 23–32.

104. Vancevska A, Nikolic A, Bonaci-Nikolic B, *et al*. (2016) Assessment of deoxyribonuclease activity in serum samples of patients with systemic lupus erythematosus: fluorescence-based method versus ELISA. *J Clin Lab Anal* **30**(6): 797–803.

105. Skiljevic D, Jeremic I, Nikolic M, *et al*. (2013) Serum DNase I activity in systemic lupus erythematosus: correlation with immunoserological markers, the disease activity and organ involvement. *Clin Chem Lab Med* **51**: 1083–1091.

106. Velders M, Treff G, Machus K, *et al*. (2014) Exercise is a potent stimulus for enhancing circulating DNase activity. *Clin Biochem* **47**: 471–474.

107. Sato S, Takenaka S. (2014) Highly sensitive nuclease assays based on chemically modified DNA or RNA. *Sensors* **14**: 12437–12450.

108. Choi SJ, Szoka FC. (2000) Fluorometric determination of deoxyribonuclease I activity with PicoGreen. *Anal Biochem* **281**: 95–97.

109. Macanovic M, Lachmann PJ. (1997) Measurement of deoxyribonuclease I (DNase) in the serum and urine of systemic lupus erythematosus (SLE)-prone NZB/NZW mice by a new radial enzyme diffusion assay. *Clin Exper Immunol* **108**: 220–226.

110. Trubetskoy VS, Hagstrom JE, Budker VG. (2002) Self-quenched covalent fluorescent dye-nucleic acid conjugates as polymeric substrates for enzymatic nuclease assays. *Anal Biochem* **300**: 22–26.

111. Sonawane S, Khanolkar V, Namavari A, *et al.* (2012) Ocular surface extracellular DNA and nuclease activity imbalance: a new paradigm for inflammation in dry eye disease. *Invest Ophthalmol Visual Sci* **53**: 8253–8263.

112. Kiedrowski MR, Kavanaugh JS, Malone CL, *et al.* (2011) Nuclease modulates biofilm formation in community-associated methicillin-resistant Staphylococcus aureus. *PloS One* **6**: e26714.

113. Barra GB, Santa Rita TH, de Almeida Vasques J, *et al.* (2015) EDTA-mediated inhibition of DNases protects circulating cell-free DNA from *ex vivo* degradation in blood samples. *Clin Biochem* **48**: 976–981.

114. Barra GB, Silva VM, Jácomo RH, *et al.* (2014) Sodium citrate at 8% is equivalent to EDTA as anticoagulant of choice for circulating cell-free DNA analysis: low contamination by blood cells genomic DNA and inhibition of blood nuclease activity. *Clin Chem* **60**: S190.

115. El Messaoudi S, Rolet F, Mouliere F, Thierry AR. (2013) Circulating cell free DNA: preanalytical considerations. *Clin Chim Acta* **424**: 222–230.

116. Mann KG, Whelihan MF, Butenas S, Orfeo T. (2007) Citrate anticoagulation and the dynamics of thrombin generation. *J Thromb Haemost* **5**: 2055–2061.

117. Lee G, Arepally GM. (2012) Anticoagulation techniques in apheresis: from heparin to citrate and beyond. *J Clin Apheresis* **27**: 117–125.

118. Gray E, Hogwood J, Mulloy B. (2012) The anticoagulant and antithrombotic mechanisms of heparin. *Handb Exper Pharmacol* (207): 43–61.

119. Adachi I, Iwaki H, Adachi H, *et al.* (1986) Heparin-induced leukocyte lysis *in vitro*. *J Pharmacobio Dyn* **9**: 207–210.

120. Santa Rita TH, Jácomo RH, Abdalla LF, *et al.* (2015) Enrichment of genomic DNA amount in serum by transport and storage at ambient temperature makes it an alternative matrix for molecular assays: high-yield of DNA, automated DNA extraction- friendly and direct use as template in qPCR. *Clin Chem* **61**: S176.

121. Clinical and Laboratory Standards Institute. *Tubes and Additives for Venous and Capillary Blood Specimen Collection: Approved Standard*, 6th ed. Clinical and Laboratory Standards Institute, 2010.

Chapter 8

Isolating Circulating Exosomes as Biomarkers: Challenges and Opportunities

Alexander Semaan and Anirban Maitra

Abstract

In addition to free extracellular DNA, blood plasma also contains nucleic acids encased in vesicles with lipid bilayer membranes. These can be divided into exosomes and extracellular vesicles, and although the two types overlap in some markers and physical properties, they are generated by different mechanisms. Exosomes can be actively secreted from cells, including cancer cells, and the stability of their cargo makes them a promising source of biomarker targets. In this chapter, we describe the origins, isolation strategies, nucleic acid content, and biomarker potential of exosomes.

Extracellular Vesicle Properties and Nomenclature

Extracellular vesicles (EV) are a heterogeneous class of cell-derived membranous particles with a storied history. Initially, these membranous particles were described as "garbage bins" of living or dying cells and received limited attention.[1] In the early 1980s two groups independently reported the discovery of what today is termed "exosomes", and since then, the interest in these vesicles has increased significantly.[2,3]

There is much confusion and even contradictory definitions of exosomes and other vesicles within the literature, which is due to the heterogeneity of the EV population.[4] It is important to stress the presence of two distinct EV types that differ by origin, biological and pathological function, and size. Although the presented classification is an oversimplification, it reflects the current state of knowledge and is based on the recommendations of the International Society for Extracellular Vesicles (ISEV). With that said, it is possible that the current stated classification system will change or expand in the future based on ongoing studies.

1. Exosomes (size: 50–150 nm, buoyant density: 1.11–1.19 g/mL), also known as nanovesicles or dexosomes. The term "exosome" was first introduced by Johnstone *et al.* in 1987 with the description of intraluminal vesicles (ILV).[1] Biogenesis of these particles is through inward budding of the endomembrane system into the multivesicular endosome (MVE) by fission of cytosol. After additional cargo loading and maturation, they are released into the extracellular space upon fusion of MVEs with the cellular lipid membrane and termed exosomes.[2,3] Exosomes have crucial functions in multiple physiological and pathological processes including cell–cell communication, inflammation, stem cell expansion, and tumorigenesis,[5] and are detectable in nearly all body fluids including blood, saliva, urine, breast milk, amniotic fluid, and ascites. Importantly, the exosomal cargo composition varies greatly and includes proteins, liquids, and nucleic acids. The diversity of exosomal content and its

modification based on the conditions of the cell of origin points to a highly selective loading of exosomal cargo depending on the physiological or pathological state.[6]

2. EV (size: 50 nm up to 1000 nm, buoyant density: undefined), also known as apoptotic bodies, microparticles, microvesicles, blebbing vesicles, and oncosomes. In contrast to the production of exosomes within the endosomal system, microvesicles are formed by ectocytosis. This process involves the outward budding and fission of the cellular membrane to form secreted particles.[7] Currently there is no clear subclassification of EV, which is mainly due to the fact that nobody knows how many functionally distinct subtypes exist. There are substantial efforts ongoing to close this gap in knowledge and characterize the heterogenous nature of EVs.[8,9]

Although of distinct origin, both vesicle types share common intracellular mechanisms and sorting machineries, leading to significant overlap in membrane bound components and cargo. As has been confirmed by reports investigating overlapping subgroups of vesicles after isolation, the two populations are not completely distinguishable by ultracentrifugation and density gradient isolation techniques based on their physical properties (size, density).[10] Additionally, many details in key biogenesis functions are still waiting to be revealed. This chapter will focus on the role, cargo, and isolation methods of exosomes.

Exosomal Function and Biomarker Potential

Once discounted as garbage bins of cells, exosomes have experienced a renaissance over the last decades. Research into exosomes and other vesicles has gained traction as we begin to understand how they play a crucial role in cell–cell communication to orchestrate multiple physiological functions, including immune signaling, angiogenesis, aging, differentiation, and proliferation.[11–13] In particular, their ability to transfer genetically encoded messages has garnered attention, because for decades, intercellular communication was thought to be only possible in a paracrine, endocrine, and neuronal manner or by direct contact between cells.

Given their role in cell–cell communication, the presence of an "exosomal fingerprint" as related to disease-specific cargo may be used as biomarker for detection, surveillance, prognosis, and therapy guidance in multiple cancer types.[14] Exosomes, together with circulating tumor cells (CTC) and circulating cell-free DNA (cirDNA), are part of a new approach to tumor characterization known as "liquid biopsies."[15] In comparison to invasive tissue biopsies, blood draws can be used to help monitor treatment response, drug resistance, predict recurrence, and also serve as auxiliary staging and diagnostic markers.[16,17] EV and exosomes contain a myriad of tumor-derived molecules that reflect, in real time, the current state of the releasing cell. In contrast to fragmented cirDNA and CTCs, accumulating evidence suggests exosomal cargo is superior as a clinical biomarker in a variety of diseases.[18–20] This may be due to the cargo's protection by the lipid bilayer, as well as a higher concentration of nucleic acid copies due to selective exosomal loading.[17]

In the context of clinical utility, a urine exosome gene expression assay together with standard-of-care (SOC) tests including PSA levels, age, race, and family history was able to reliably distinguish ≥7 Gleason from low-grade prostate tumors or benign disease. These results suggest the potential for auxiliary exosomal disease staging to help guide personalized therapies and protect patients from harmful over- or undertreatment.[21] Another example of the use of exosomes in treatment monitoring was shown recently by

Bernard *et al.* The authors demonstrated in a longitudinal cohort of over 36 patients with pancreatic ductal adenocarcinoma that an increase in mutational *KRAS* burden within exosomes, but not ctDNA *KRAS* level, during therapy is associated with disease progression.[20] Especially promising is the potential identification of targetable mutations within liquid biopsies for patient stratification in the context of personalized medicine. Herein, researchers have been able to detect clinically actionable *BRAF V600E* mutations in patients,[22] as well as changes in the exosomal cargo from melanoma cell lines and patient-derived xenografts after treatment with the BRAF inhibitor Vemurafenib.[23] Additionally, *EGFR* L858R and T790M mutations from lung cancer–derived exosomes, which represent susceptible genotypes to tyrosine kinase inhibitors, have been found with higher sensitivity within exosomes compared to cirDNA.[24]

Exosomes have also been shown to provide a scaffold for enrichment of tumor-specific material in circulation by exploiting the protein surfaceome of these vesicles. Enrichment of exosomes leads to greater sensitivity of mutant detection, facilitating molecular profiling of emerging mechanisms of resistance.[25] The ability to modify and engineer exosomal cargo is also currently being evaluated as an immune-inert treatment vehicle for targeted drug delivery and immunotherapeutic approach.[15,16]

Following Peter Paget's "soil and seed" theory, exosomes have also been described as mediators of the so-called "pre-metastatic niche" formation. Herein, these vesicles have been shown to transport essential tumor-secreted factors to prime stromal tissue at distant organ sites for the outgrowth of CTC.[26]

It is also important to note that exosomes have major roles outside of tumorigenesis, including neurodegenerative and cardiovascular diseases.[27] Exosomes secreted physiologically by certain cell populations might harbor important immunomodulatory and cytoprotective properties derived from their releasing cells. For example, microvesicles released by mesenchymal stem cells (MSCs) have been shown to have a function in tissue repair and are currently being evaluated for their role in regenerative medicine.[28] Particularly in myocardial infarction (MI), there is increasing evidence of a possible protective role of purified exosomes, for example, embryonic stem cell–derived MSC exosomes in animal models of MI.[29,30] Many other pathophysiological mechanisms, like deposition of Tau protein in early Alzheimer disease, have been thought to occur via exosomal release, although no effective treatment strategy targeting this deposition has been proposed.[31,32] In contrast, memory and educational effects of exosomes in immune cells have been already used to prime organisms for future infections,[32] which is a promising strategy to protect organisms from multidrug-resistant bacteria infections.

Exosomal Biogenesis and Regulation

Regulation of exosomal biogenesis and cargo loading is a complex and not yet fully understood process that involves multiple distinct pathways.[33] It should be noted that though EV and exosomes originate from different parts of the cell, they share some common intracellular mechanisms.[34] Exosomal biogenesis may be split into three separate steps: (1) formation of ILV within MVE; (2) further maturation and transport to the cell membrane, and (3) fusion of MVEs and release of exosomes (Fig. 1). It remains unclear if cells form a single, or multiple types, MVE. Some research points to the fact that only certain MVE subpopulations have the ability to fuse with the cell membrane, while others are directed to lysosomes.[35]

An important step in the formation of ILV comprises the clustering of lipids and membrane-associated proteins in membrane

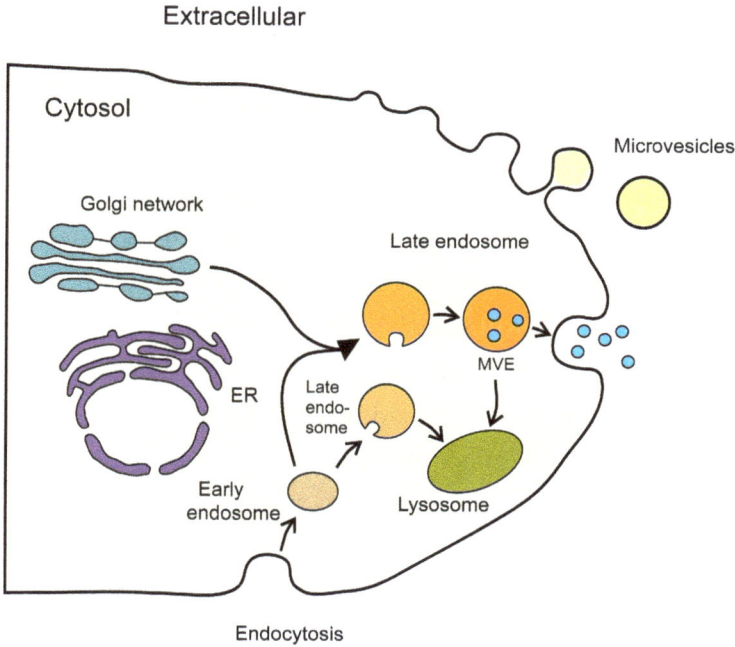

Fig. 1: Pathways of exosomal biogenesis. ER — endoplasmic reticulum; MVB — multivesicular endosome.

microdomains. This process can happen in an Endosomal Sorting Complex Required for Transport (ESCRT)-dependent or ESCRT-independent manner.[36,37] The former requires a cascade of ESCRT complexes to aggregate transmembrane cargo followed by inward budding and fission of early exosomes or ILVs. Detailed knockout studies targeting 23 ESCRT-related proteins revealed a complex synergy within the ESCRT machinery, which consists of four major complexes associated with AAA ATPase Vps4 complex.[38] Apart from ILV formation, the ESCRT has also been shown to control sorting of ubiquitinated proteins into ILVs. Details on the regulation of exosome loading, ESCRT machinery, and their related proteins, such syntenin and the syndecans, have been previously published.[39–42]

ESCRT-independent exosome formation on the other hand requires either the formation of ceramides by hydrolyzation of sphingomyelin[43] or a process that involves proteins of the tetraspanin family (e.g., CD63, CD9, and CD81) that are abundantly expressed on exosomes.[44] Exosome formation may also result from co-sorting with certain protein classes such as chaperones including heat shock 70 kDa protein (HSP70 and HSP71)[45] or lipid rafts harboring glycosylphosphatidylinositol (GPI)-anchored proteins.[46]

In summary, exosomal biogenesis is a complex, cell, and cargo-specific process influenced by multiple physiological, developmental, and pathological processes.

Exosomal Cargo

Protected by a characteristic bilipid layer, exosomal cargo is shielded from degradation in the extracellular space and blood stream. Exosomes may contain a large variety of different molecules, often mirroring the current state of their releasing cell.[35,36] The cargo is either processed from within the cells in the Golgi apparatus or upon internalization from the plasma membrane, finally leading to the formation of ILV. The exosomal content comprises membrane bound and soluble proteins, lipids, carbohydrates, and nucleic acids[47] (Fig. 2). The following section focuses on exosomal nucleic acids; details on exosomal protein content have been published previously.[48]

Nucleic Acids in Exosomes

Nucleic acids in exosomes include transcriptomic and intact mRNAs, mRNA fragments, noncoding RNA (lnRNA, snRNA, siRNA, piRNA, ncRNA, and miRNA) as well as single- or double-stranded DNA.[11,39] In contrast to cellular RNA, exosomal

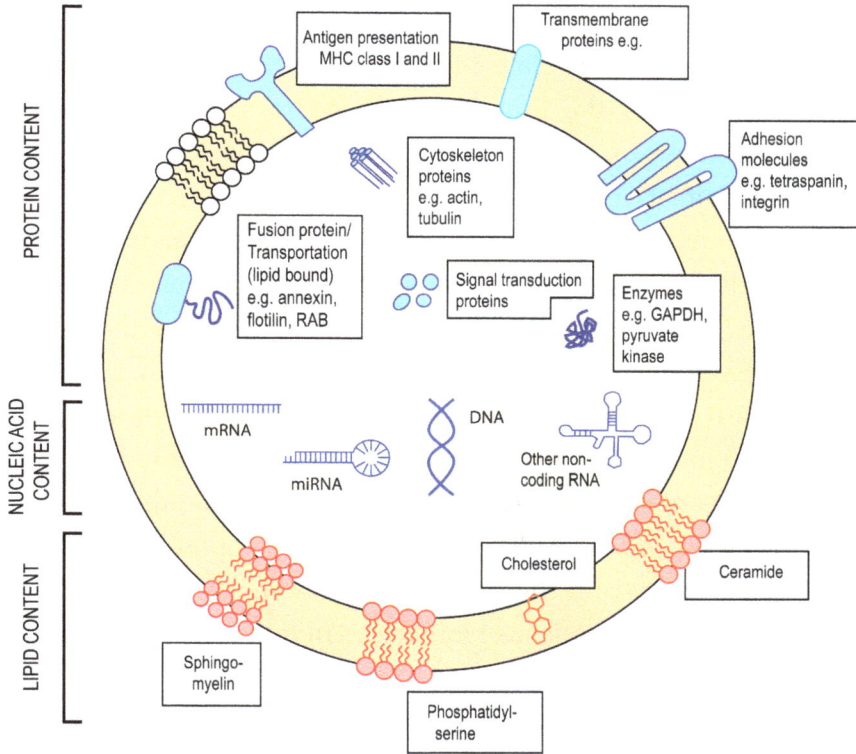

Fig. 2:   Exosomal cargo includes protein content, nucleic acid content, and lipid content.

RNA (exoRNA) is mostly devoid of the large and small ribosomal RNA subunits, which are often used for validation in cellular RNA assays.[49] In general, RNA cargo differs based on the cells of origin and their homeostatic state. In particular, cell-specific exosomal microRNA has been characterized as "fingerprints," where shifts in composition can occur in cases of disease, infection, and cancer.[26,50–53] Besides the aforementioned pathologic shifts, there have also been reports of gender-specific expression patterns for microRNA in urine-derived exosomes.[54] In general, exoRNA is more fragmented (typically <700 nucleotides) than intracellular

RNA (400–12,000 nucleotides).[55] The exact cause of this is not known, but it may be related to the RNA interference machinery within or after the formation of exosomes, RNA degeneration within the exosomes, or artificial changes upon isolation and downstream analysis.

In comparison to other extracellular nucleic acids, such as cirDNA, that is present as fragmented DNA in circulation (~170 base pairs), exosomal DNA is preserved as significantly longer lengths. Even high–molecular weight DNA has been found in plasma-derived exosomes, representing the entire genome, and mirrors the mutational status of parental cells.[22,56] There have also been reports of high-quality, double-stranded genomic DNA in exosomes isolated from cell lines and human samples by ultracentrifugation.[57] Based on these findings, exosomal DNA and RNA harbor immense potential as biomarkers in many diseases.

Selective RNA Loading into Exosomes

The specific exosomal cargo content unique to certain cell types suggests an active RNA loading and selection process based on physiologic conditions.[58,59] Several mechanisms have been proposed for this selective loading. Exosomal microRNA expresses a distinct EXOmotif (GGAG tetranucleotide) and harbors a consensus sequence within the 3'UTR end (25nt sequence, which contains a short CTGCC core domain on a stem-loop structure and carries a miR-1289-binding site). Both of these motifs may act as "zip codes" for intracellular loading into exosomes.[60,61] Additionally, different machineries have been implicated in exosomal RNA sorting including the ESCRT-II complex, tetraspanin-enriched microdomains, ceramides, protein argonaute-2 (AGO2) and microRNA-induced silencing complex (mRISC).[62,63] Finally, it is also important to note that cellular RNA levels and their availability will directly affect exosomal RNA loading.[64]

Measurement of Exosomal RNA Quantity and Quality

As RNA is intrinsically unstable, particularly in the presence of external factors (e.g., heat, mechanical forces, UV light, and RNases), and since exosomal RNA in itself is already largely fragmented, it is important to follow stringent laboratory techniques when conducting RNA-based research. This includes use of RNase-free working areas and reagents (chemical or mechanical inactivation of RNase prior to use), and working on ice and in a time-efficient manner for sample processing. To effectively quantify the low concentration of exosomal nucleic acids, it is necessary to rule out extravesicular contamination. This involves treating isolated exosomes with RNases before exosomal lysis in order to degrade extra-exosomal soluble or protein-bound nucleic acids. While extracellular RNA will be degraded, intravesicle cargo is protected by the lipid bilayer. In addition to the removal of any extravesicular RNAs, RNase treatment also helps to resolve exosomal aggregation and increase yield.[65] In the case of potential protein contamination (e.g., cell lines cultured with protein-rich media), addition of proteinase-K before exosomal lysis releases any protein-bound RNA and reduces protein and protein-bound RNA contamination.[66]

Quantification of exosomal nucleic acid levels remains challenging, but with increasing sensitivity of commercial detection systems, it is becoming more manageable. Traditional spectrophotometer devices like Nanodrop are typically insufficiently sensitive to reliably quantify exoRNA concentrations. Fluorometer devices like Qubit have a lower limit of detection for nucleic acids (down to 0.25 ng RNA/µl) and are able to distinguish between RNA and DNA, thus also allowing digital elimination of DNA contamination. Another option for exoRNA quantification involves utilizing a Bioanalyzer Pico Chip, which is able to detect concentrations down to 50 pg/µL. Importantly, the Bioanalyzer provides an electrophoresis-like virtual RNA size profile, which also helps to visually confirm the presence of different-sized nucleic acids.[67] It has to be noted that quality control of RNA on the Bioanalyzer is often based on the large ribosomal subunits (18S and 28S) that are often nonexistent in exoRNA samples. As the quality of RNA cannot be measured, some reports suggest that the system may be error-prone based on vulnerability to salt concentration in the sample, ladder variability, and co-detection of contaminating DNA.[68] Among the most sensitive methods, real-time PCR has the ability to detect quantities of RNA down to 1 fg. Though incredibly precise, one has to bear in mind that this technique is sensitive to DNA contamination. Detailed comparison of different RNA quantification methods has been previously described.[69]

Depending on the intended downstream analysis, several issues must be kept in mind to minimize potential bias. Sources of bias that especially affect high throughput techniques are summarized in the following. First, the extraction methodology may impact the final RNA composition. For example, TRIzol tends to concentrate strong anti-GC content especially in small RNA amounts, as highly structured small RNAs or those with low GC content are less efficient in interacting with carrier.[70] Also, different NGS library preparation kits might affect exoRNA sequencing results by variation in adaptor ligation or hybridization,[71] although novel strategies have been developed to tackle this obstacle. Additionally, some kits favor either smaller or larger RNA fragments that might lead to an underrepresentation of "mid-size" RNA fragments in the final library pool. The sequencing platform itself, and subsequent bioinformatics processing of the sequencing data (e.g., mapping order to multiple databases), also has an impact on RNA sequencing results through various parameters (for details see[72]). None of the current library processing or analysis methods are completely unbiased, which renders it necessary to perform an orthogonal method of validation, e.g., by RT-qPCR and normalization of data.

In comparison to mRNA, small RNAs, such as microRNAs, are relatively stable. Their abundance within exosomes and their function as regulators of posttranscriptional gene expression[73] make microRNAs attractive candidates as cancer biomarkers. There is also an increasing body of evidence for functional cell-to-cell transfer of miRNAs via exosomes, adding to their roles in tumorigenesis.[64,74] There are currently various commercial kits available for isolation of exosomal microRNA from primary cultures as well as patient biofluids.

Exosomal Identification

Based on the increasing significance of exosomes in health and disease, multiple principles and guidelines for exosome detection have been established, for example, the position statement from the ISEV.[75] It is always recommended to run all experiments with appropriate positive and negative control samples to identify systemic errors and sources of contamination. Additionally, guidelines recommend the use of different methods of exosome verification. The gold standard for exosomal imaging is transmission electron microscopy (TEM). Preparations require fixation, embedding, cutting, and staining, which results in a collapsed artifactual cup-shaped structure. TEM also allows for reliable size measurements of EV, and specific subpopulations can be identified through immuno-gold-labelling. Standard views should comprise wide field view as well as close-ups of single vesicles.[75] Another method for exosome identification is flow-cytometry. As exosomes are too small in size to be reliably detected through flow cytometry, vesicles are typically captured onto large particles or beads and then fluorescently tagged with antibodies of interest including CD63 or CD9.[76]

Another popular method of exosome detection is through nanoparticle tracking analysis (NTA).[77] This technique measures size distribution and vesicle concentration based on their Brownian motion with a dark field microscope, although size distributions should be validated with values calculated through TEM.[78,79] NTA is not able to differentiate nonvesicular particles such as protein aggregates with overlapping size distributions of vesicles but is superior in size measurements compared to dynamic light scattering.[80] Another method for characterization of single vesicles is known as resistive pulse sensing (RPS), which is based on the Coulter principle and tracks size and concentration of nanoparticles passing through pores of a stationary phase.[81] Similar to NTA, RPS is not capable of distinguishing between nonvesicular and vesicular particles.

Besides identification based on their physical properties, isolation of exosomes after enrichment is often verified by Western blot, ELISA, or proteomic analysis in order to demonstrate the presence of abundantly expressed exosomal-specific proteins. Thanks to evolving isolation and analytical technologies, the list of new exosomal protein content is constantly growing. As of July 2018, a total of around 7500 different proteins have been described, but only 500 of them account for approximately 90% of exosomal proteins.[82] The general characterization of exosomes is typically done by using at least three exosomal markers (described in the following).[74,75] Additionally, the ISEV recommends confirming the under-representation or absence of intracellular proteins associated with compartments other than the plasma membrane or endosomes, and comparing protein composition of the isolated exosomal fraction with supernatant and negative controls. Protein analysis is ideally performed by Western blot, FACS, or global proteomic analysis using mass spectrometry techniques in a semi-quantitative assay.[75]

The most commonly used markers for exosome identification are the tetraspanin family members CD9, CD63, and CD81. More recent reports have also identified them to be abundantly expressed in apoptotic bodies and microvesicles.[83] Based on the cargo sorting machinery involved in their biogenesis, ESCRT components such as ALG-2-interacting protein X (ALIX) and tumor susceptibility gene 101 protein (TSG101) can also be identified, but these are not specific to exosomes.[84] Some papers indicate a lack of commonly used markers in certain subpopulations of exosome such as small vesicles. For example, Kowal *et al.* identified certain subcategories of small vesicles/exosomes that lack bona fide exosomal markers CD9 and CD63, which suggests that their biogenesis does not involve the endosomal pathway.[5] In contrast, all small vesicles with the size of exosomes have shown abundant expression in Annexin XI, ADAM10, ACE, and EHD4. These results are consistent with other recent proteomic characterizations of EV and exosomes from platelets and tumor cells[85–87] and might point to the fact that these markers represent higher accuracy for exosomal isolation. In summary, after exclusion of larger vesicles by isolation techniques, CD63 might be one of the best markers to pull down or identify endosome-derived exosomes, although some cell types do secrete CD63-devoid vesicles.[87–89]

Other markers have been proposed, which are described as more cancer specific. For example, similar to the field of CTC, the use of EPCAM antibodies has been reported as a specific method to isolate tumor exosomes from epithelial carcinomas.[90] More recently, we have shown that CLDN4, EPCAM, CD151, LGALS3BP, HIST2H2BE, and HIST2H2BF can specifically isolate exosomes from pancreatic ductal adenocarcinoma. Biofluid specificity has also been reported with regard to exosomal surface marker repertoire, whereby lectin-abundant exosomes have been identified in patient-derived urine samples.[91]

Exosomal Isolation Strategies

The first step in the successful isolation of EV is to optimize the collection conditions of the starting fluid. If working with exosomes from cell culture supernatant, contamination of the supernatant with other sources of extracellular exosomes such as fetal bovine serum (FBS) has to be minimized or at the very least taken into consideration in downstream analysis.[92]

If the starting material comprises biofluids such as mammalian whole blood, precautions should be taken to prevent platelet activation.[93,94] This is typically done through the use of anticoagulants in blood collection tubes; however, it is important to know that anticoagulants may impair downstream analysis, specifically PCR inhibition by heparin.[95] As blood is one of the most commonly used sources of exosomes, standardization of blood collection and processing is of upmost importance. For example, prolonged stasis using tourniquets should be avoided to prevent hemolysis,[96] patient volume status should be taken into account, and even circadian rhythms have been shown to have an impact in the context of liquid biopsy analysis. Other pre-analytical variables to consider are standardization of needle diameter as well as the need to discard the first 2 mL of blood collected to avoid contamination with non-blood cells.[97] Few reports exist comparing the exosomal fraction derived from human serum versus plasma, but as serum is highly influenced by the coagulation system, plasma is typically considered the preferred source for exosomal isolation. Among blood collection tubes, acid citrate dextrose (ACD) tubes have been reported to be superior because of their impairment of platelet exosome formation.[98] Handling of the blood vials is also important for exosomal quality. Exosomal yields are maximized with gentle handling and fast processing after collection, usually within 4 hr.[99] To minimize the number of white and red blood cells, as well as platelets, that might release exosomes upon activation, plasma is separated from whole blood. Room temperature, two-step centrifugation (2×15 min, 2500g) with lowest deceleration settings is recommended for plasma isolation. Plasma collection should also stop approximately 5 mm above the buffy coat meniscus.[100] It is also important to consider the short- and long-term storage of collected samples, where snap freezing of aliquots has been recommended for exosome storage. There is a limited amount of studies investigating the potential impact of long-term freezing on the recovery, morphology, and impact on downstream analysis. In general, fresh processing of isolated exosomal pellet provides the best yield, whereas extended freezer storage of exosomes may increase their size and change their physical properties, such as their repertoire of surface proteins. These morphological changes are due to an expansion of ice crystals in the spherical lipid bilayer and consequent membrane disruption, which may ultimately lead to membrane fusion of neighboring vesicles.[101] Nonetheless, storage temperatures of –70°C to –80°C are recommended over higher temperature (–20°C to –60°C) for long-term storage.[102]

Herein, we will describe six current strategies for exosome isolation. These are either based on different physical properties of the vesicles (e.g., size, density, shape) or on the capture of exosomes by specific molecules that are abundantly expressed on their surface. All have their own advantages and disadvantages and have to be tailored and optimized based on specific needs (Fig. 3).

Ultracentrifugation

Ultracentrifugation (Fig. 3a) uses centrifugal forces to separate particles in suspension based on their density, size, and shape, as well as the density and viscosity of the solvent. Ultracentrifugation applies exceptionally high centrifugal forces of up to 100,000g to isolate nanosized vesicles of interest and is still considered the gold standard for exosome purification. Due to its long-term cost efficiency and relative purity of extraction, this technique is used by many of the laboratories studying exosome biology,[103] although the initial capital expense is high. Nonetheless, it is important to highlight that different equipment (e.g., rotor type and diameter) and isolation parameters like centrifugation time and speed produce significantly different populations of exosomes with specific protein and RNA content.[104,105]

Usually sequential ultracentrifugation steps with increasing gravitational ("g") speeds are carried out in order to eliminate cellular debris and isolate EV of a desired size. Exosomal purity can be increased by combining density gradient separation with ultracentrifugation. This also allows the separation of low-density exosomes from high-density protein aggregates, which are often a source of contamination from differential ultracentrifugation.[106] There are two major subtypes of density-gradient centrifugation (Fig. 3b). Isopycnic centrifugation sediments particles based on their density profile to a defined equilibrium position (equilibrium of density)

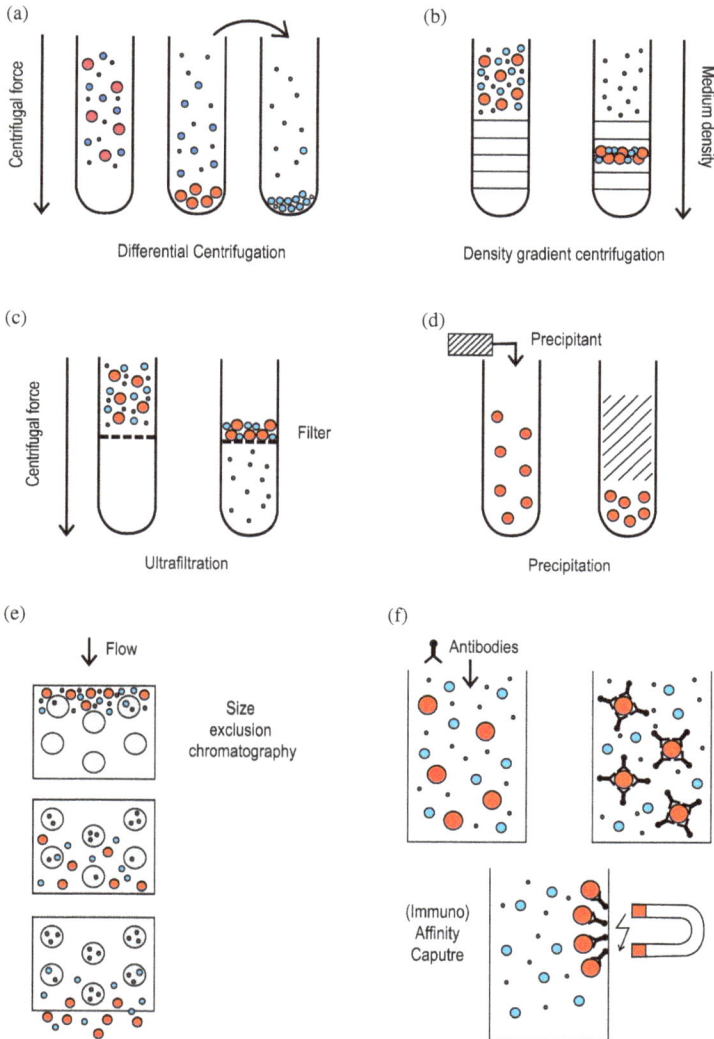

Fig. 3: Strategies for exosome purification: (a) differential centrifugation, (b) density gradient centrifugation, (c) ultrafiltration, (d) precipitation, (e) size exclusion chromatography, (f) affinity capture.

but needs high centrifugation speed and a long running time. The isopycnic position is 1.10–1.21 g/mL in case of the commonly used solvent cesium chloride.[107] In contrast, moving-zone ultracentrifugation uses differences in the molecular weight (size and mass) for separation. Although moving-zone ultracentrifugation allows for the separation of vesicles with different sizes but similar densities, it is important to mention that centrifugation time directly affects the position of the exosomal fraction within the density gradient, which therefore needs to be controlled rigorously. Insufficient centrifugation time will result in an incomplete separation, whereas excess centrifugation time will co-precipitate all analytes. Additionally, loading volumes are very limited, which restricts a high through put.

Ultrafiltration

This technique uses exosomal size, deformation capability, and molecular weight to selectively pass them through a membrane filter with defined exclusion limits (Fig. 3c). The biggest advantage of ultrafiltration is the ease of use, the short processing time, and the low cost per sample. On the other hand, the filtration process may result in possible deformation of vesicles and the loss of specificity in isolating exosomal fractions. This technique is of particular use in cell-free samples like urine where researchers have shown similar efficiency of vesicle isolation compared to much more time-consuming protocols like ultracentrifugation.[108] For suspensions with a high cellular content, removal of large cells and particles has to be performed prior to ultrafiltration. Yield may be affected by clogging or vesicle trapping on the membranes.[109]

Polyethylene Glycol (PEG) Precipitation

Polyethylene glycol (PEG) precipitation (Fig. 3d) uses exosomal solubility and dispersal properties to isolate them from a suspension. The technique requires a hydrophilic polymer (e.g., PEG), which binds water molecules and forces hydrophobic contents to settle. The precipitate itself is usually generated from pre-processed samples (removal of cells, cell fragments, and debris by centrifugation) upon an incubation step at 4°C followed by centrifugation or filtration for harvesting the precipitate. The workflow is easy to handle, cost efficient, does not require specialized equipment and is easily scalable to sample size.[110] Nonetheless, exosomes are not exclusively precipitated, and the background of hydrophobic molecules and particles — especially co-precipitating proteins — can be high.[111] Also, precipitating conditions must be optimized to different viscosity levels of samples, leading to the requirement for pre- and post-precipitation cleaning steps.

Size Exclusion Chromatography (SEC)

Size exclusion chromatography (SEC) (Fig. 3e) uses the hydrodynamic volume of particles for their separation and can be used for low-volume samples. Despite its name, SEC uses not only the size of the particle for separation but also their varying diffusion volumes over a stationary porous phase. This is one of its main differences from techniques like ultrafiltration that separate particles based solely on their physical size. Upon entering the stationary polymer layer with micron-scale polymer beads containing pores of different sizes, smaller particles experience a leap in their available diffusion volume leading to a prolonged retention time. In contrast, larger particles with a smaller available diffusion volume are quickly forced out of the porous layer in the isolation column. Thus, larger particles elute faster through the stationary polymer compared to smaller molecules. A big advantage of SEC is its resulting high purity of exosomes and data reproducibility. Unfortunately, it's a time-consuming technique that requires specialized technical expertise and equipment. A possible source of contamination to consider in SEC is the co-isolation of lipoproteins (high- and low-density lipoproteins and chylomicrons) that show similar diffusion volumes to exosomes.

Immunoprecipitation/Microfluidics Devices

Immunoaffinity-based separation assays (Fig. 3f) use exosomal antigens to capture vesicles. A basic requirement for the use of any immunoprecipitation is the presence of a unique, membrane-bound antigen that is expressed at a significant concentration on the outer lipid layer of exosomes. Herein, one might rely on "general" exosomal identification markers (e.g., CD9, TSG101, or CD69) or target cancer–specific molecules. Preferably, no soluble counterpart of these molecules should exist, in order to prevent unintended and uncontrolled binding. The most commonly used separation technique is magnetic pull-down, where magnetic beads are coated with specific antibodies with a high affinity for the desired exosomal antigen. The bound vesicles can then be either directly lysed to discharge their content or released from the beads for further downstream analysis (see section "Exosomal identification" for details on the exosomal antigens).

Other methods use microfluidics devices that exploit membrane-coated immunoprecipitation on a chip.[112] These devices provide an efficient method for exosomal isolation from low-volume samples. Some systems also allow the on-chip integration of exosomal characterization and nucleic acid extraction. For example, ExoChip uses anti-CD63 IgG antibodies to capture exosomes, quantifies the number of captured exosomes after fluorescent carbocyanine dye (DiO, 3,3′-Dioctadecyloxacarbocyanine Perchlorate) staining with a plate reader, and enables downstream isolation of intact exosomal RNA.[113] With advancing production capacity and more precise manufacturing, microfluidics devices promise a more efficient, time-saving, and cost-effective approach to isolate exosomes that is consolidated on a single chip, although it has to be mentioned that to date, no system meets the stringent criteria required in a clinical trial setting. Immunoaffinity capture methods result in highly purified exosomal fractions but at the cost of lower exosomal yields. This is due to the fact that one is limited in isolating the specific exosomal phenotype of interest. Additionally, it is important to note that exosomes may aggregate or be shielded by protein or platelet coating, resulting in a reduced binding to antibodies.

Field Flow Fractionation

In contrast to classical chromatography, field flow fractionation (FFF) uses differences in particle diffusion capabilities to separate particles in a long narrow channel. Exosomes in solution are pumped through this chamber with a continuous parabolic flow. In a separation zone this continuous flow is exposed to a crossfield comprised of a perpendicular force, for example, electric charges, magnetism, light or gravity. This interaction between the parabolic flow and the perpendicular force separates exosomes based on the Brownian motion of particles. In contrast to classical chromatographs, smaller particles like exosomes are separated early creating a reversed eluate profile.[114] In addition to classical FFF, other separation forces such as acoustic nanofilters using ultrasonic waves have been described as a strategy in exosome isolation, which allows for versatile size selection of vesicles.[115]

Various commercial kits for the direct isolation of stable exosomal microRNAs have been released. In principle, exosomes are isolated in a first step on a membrane filter. Following lysis, exosomal microRNA content is purified in a column through a consecutive protocol of washing solutions. Many of these isolation kits are popular because they are time efficient and user friendly, but it is important to stress that most of the kits produce a high exosomal yield but also suffer from a relatively high albumin contamination. For detailed comparison of different performance of kits, please refer to the technique comparison in the following section, as well as to other studies.[67,116,117]

All of these methods carry advantages and disadvantages, and ultimately it is the user's decision as to which strategy provides the most effective means of answering the biological question of interest. Combining different isolation principles may be a powerful tool to minimize contamination and achieve a high purity, but is time consuming and leads to a significant decrease in yield. Several reports have been published providing valuable guidelines in identifying common pitfalls and outlining consensus findings for researchers in this field.[59,93,100] Another important source of comparison is the crowdsourcing knowledgebase that centralizes EV studies with the aim of a more standardized approach.[118]

Comparison Between Isolation Techniques

Although the choice of exosomal isolation technique has a significant impact on the findings and reproducibility of a study, there are a limited number of high-quality studies comparing the yield and quality of different isolation methods using the same input material.[119,120] In 2014, van Deun compared two commercial isolation kits ExoQuick (System Biosciences) and Total Exosome Isolation Reagent (Invitrogen) to ultracentrifugation and density gradient centrifugation (OptiPrep, Sigma Aldrich) using supernatant from a breast cancer cell line.[119] The authors showed that, based on electron microscopy and Western blot, OptiPrep density gradient centrifugation outperformed all other techniques in terms of purity, although with significantly lower yields. Similarly, Ting-Tang *et al.* compared a variety of commercial isolation methods with ultracentrifugation using cell culture media and found the highest purity, but the lowest yield, of exosomes was obtained with ultracentrifugation.[67] In 2017, Helwa *et al.* compared different volumes of noncancerous human serum processed with four different exosome isolation methodologies: miRCURY (Exiqon), ExoQuick (System Biosciences), Total Exosome Isolation Reagent (Invitrogen), and ultracentrifugation.[117] The authors used NTA, Western blot analysis (for CD9 and CD63), TEM, and droplet digital PCR to confirm exosomal isolation and compare yields. They concluded that the commercial kits provide higher yields for most input volumes, although no evaluation of contamination in the exosome isolates was carried out. In general, commercial kits have shown up to 100-fold higher RNA yield but with accompanying higher contamination of soluble proteins. Other studies have shown superior purification when using immunoaffinity-based approaches compared to density gradient ultracentrifugation.[121,122] In summary, there exists a tradeoff between exosomal purity and yield, which must be adapted to the needs of the study.

Artifacts

Though exciting new results have been presented over the last decade in the field of EV, exosomal research is still heavily prone to bias and artifacts. This stems from the fact that there is no uniform definition of exosomes and other EV subtypes. This nonstringent terminology across published articles leads to overlapping definitions of vesicle subpopulations.[33] It is also important to keep in mind that most vesicles isolated from human blood originate from healthy cells. The mean EV concentration in healthy individuals reaches approximately 10^7–10^9/mL blood and it needs significant technical abilities to analyze changes over this background[123] and distinguish exosomes originating from, for example, cancer cells. Herein, the problem with most published protocols for isolation of EV is their nonselective isolation of all circulating exosomes, in contrast to a cancer-specific exosomal pull-down.

Due to their small diameter and cargo load, validation of exosomal isolation is still challenging. In this context, several former proposed "exosomal markers" have been shown to be present in a wide variety of EV subtypes (e.g., major histocompatibility complex molecules, flotillins and heat shock proteins), meaning that studies that have used these likely had a heterogeneous population of vesicle types in their analysis.[8,124] Additionally, the primary isolation fluid (e.g., saliva, urine, blood, cell culture supernatant) significantly affects the possible contaminants that may be present. For example, bacteria-derived material is a source of contamination in human nasal fluid and saliva, whereas Tamm–Horsefall glycoprotein has been reported as major contaminant in human urine.[59]

Co-isolation of other soluble particles is a common source of artifacts. Physical characteristics overlapping with large proteins, protein aggregates, and lipoproteins, especially in complex human suspensions like blood, saliva, or urine, make the isolation of exosomes based on their physical properties prone to contamination.[109,125] Protein complexes and single proteins may also co-bind microRNA and therefore significantly affect downstream analysis. Another source of contamination are nonexosomal–associated forms of extracellular RNA bound to lipoprotein (HDL and LDL) complexes, ribonucleoprotein complexes (RNPs) or viral particles that might be co-isolated with exosomes.[125] Both lipoproteins, as well as postprandially increased chylomicrons, have been shown to carry nucleic acids, and their co-purification might lead to compromised results.[126,127] Specifically, each lipoprotein fraction (HDL, LDL, VLDL, and chylomicrons) has a size or buoyant density profile that overlaps with exosomes. In this context, although VLDL and chylomicrons have overlapping sizes to exosomes (≥ 60 nm), they may be separated by their different density buoyance of <1.06 g/cm^3 versus exosomal 1.11–1.19 g/cm^3 density buoyance, whereas HDL can be separated from exosomes based solely on their smaller size (10 nm vs. 50–150 nm), although they show an overlapping density buoyance.

To reliably distinguish between extravesicular and intravesicular RNA, exosomal samples should be treated with RNase and proteinase prior to exosome lysis. Herein, some reports question the presence of high–molecular weight DNA and ribosomal RNA in exosomes and ascribe their presence in exosomes to co-isolation with other molecules.[59] Like human samples, cell culture supernatant comprises its own challenges for exosomal isolation. There is, for example, concern in the exosomal community regarding the contamination of RNA results from cell culture–isolated exosomes by carryover from FBS used in culture media.[92]

Conclusions

EV, including exosomes, have experienced a renaissance over the last decade. Multiple new discoveries about their role in crucial (patho-)physiological mechanisms, as well as their highly protected cargo that shows immense potential as a source of biomarkers, resulted in a spike of interest. Despite their importance, EV isolation and characterization harbors multiple challenges and pitfalls. Following now established guidelines together with careful experimental design offer the opportunity to fully unlock their potential and integrate EV biomarkers into routine clinical workup.

References

1. Johnstone RM, Adam M, Hammond JR, Orr L, Turbide C. (1987) Vesicle formation during reticulocyte maturation. Association of plasma membrane activities with released vesicles (exosomes). *J Biol Chem* **262**: 9412–9420.

2. Pan BT, Teng K, Wu C, Adam M, Johnstone RM. (1985) Electron microscopic evidence for externalization of the transferrin receptor in vesicular form in sheep reticulocytes. *J Cell Biol* **101**: 942–948.

3. Harding C, Heuser J, Stahl P. (1984) Endocytosis and intracellular processing of transferrin and colloidal gold-transferrin in rat reticulocytes: demonstration of a pathway for receptor shedding. *Eur J Cell Biol* **35**: 256–263.

4. Gould SJ, Raposo G. (2013) As we wait: coping with an imperfect nomenclature for extracellular vesicles. *J Extracell Vesicles* **2**: 20389.

5. Cicero Lo A, Stahl PD, Raposo G. (2015) Extracellular vesicles shuffling intercellular messages: for good or for bad. *Curr Opin Cell Biol* **35**: 69–77.

6. Raposo G, Stoorvogel W. (2013) Extracellular vesicles: exosomes, microvesicles, and friends. *J Cell Biol* **200**: 373–383.

7. Tricarico C, Clancy J, D'Souza-Schorey C. (2017) Biology and biogenesis of shed microvesicles. *Small GTPases* **8**: 220–232.

8. Kowal J, Arras G, Colombo M, *et al.* (2016) Proteomic comparison defines novel markers to characterize heterogeneous populations of extracellular vesicle subtypes. *Proc Natl Acad Sci USA* **113**: E968–E977.

9. Willms E, Johansson HJ, Mäger I, *et al.* (2016) Cells release subpopulations of exosomes with distinct molecular and biological properties. *Sci Rep* **6**: 22519.

10. Shen B, Wu N, Yang J-M, Gould SJ. (2011) Protein targeting to exosomes/microvesicles by plasma membrane anchors. *J Biol Chem* **286**: 14383–14395.

11. Valadi H, Ekstr K, Bossios A, Margareta S., Lee JJ, Lötvall JO. (2007) Exosome-mediated transfer of mRNAs and microRNAs is a novel mechanism of genetic exchange between cells. *Nat Cell Biol* **9**: 654–659.

12. Robbins PD, Dorronsoro A, Booker CN. (2016) Regulation of chronic inflammatory and immune processes by extracellular vesicles. *J Clin Invest* **126**: 1173–1180.

13. Ibrahim A, Marbán E. (2016) Exosomes: fundamental biology and roles in cardiovascular physiology. *Annu Rev Physiol* **78**: 67–83.

14. Hoshino A, Costa-Silva B, Shen T-L, *et al.* (2015) Tumour exosome integrins determine organotropic metastasis. *Nature* **527**: 329–335.

15. Crowley E, Di Nicolantonio F, Loupakis F, Bardelli A. (2013) Liquid biopsy: monitoring cancer-genetics in the blood. *Nat Rev Clin Oncol* **10**: 472–484.

16. Wan JCM, Massie C, Garcia-Corbacho J, *et al.* (2017) Liquid biopsies come of age: towards implementation of circulating tumour DNA. *Nat Rev Cancer* **17**: 223–238.

17. Siravegna G, Marsoni S, Siena S, Bardelli A. (2017) Integrating liquid biopsies into the management of cancer. *Nat Rev Clin Oncol* **14**: 531–548.

18. Halvaei S, Daryani S, Eslami-S Z, *et al.* (2018) Exosomes in cancer liquid biopsy: a focus on breast cancer. *Mol Ther Nucleic Acids* **10**: 131–141.

19. Nedaeinia R, Manian M, Jazayeri MH, *et al.* (2017) Circulating exosomes and exosomal microRNAs as biomarkers in gastrointestinal cancer. *Cancer Gene Ther* **24**: 48–56.

20. Bernard V, Kim DU, San Lucas FA, *et al.* (2018) Circulating nucleic acids associate with outcomes of patients with pancreatic cancer. *Gastroenterology* **156**(1): 108–118.e4.

21. McKiernan J, Donovan MJ, O'Neill V, *et al.* (2016) A novel urine exosome gene expression assay to predict high-grade prostate cancer at initial biopsy. *JAMA Oncol* **2**: 882–889.

22. Thakur BK, Zhang H, Becker A, *et al.* (2014) Double-stranded DNA in exosomes: a novel biomarker in cancer detection. *Cell Res* **24**: 766–769.

23. Lunavat TR, Cheng L, Einarsdottir BO, *et al.* (2017) BRAFV600 inhibition alters the microRNA cargo in the vesicular secretome of malignant melanoma cells. *Proc Natl Acad Sci USA* **114**: E5930–E5939.

24. Krug AK, Enderle D, Karlovich C, *et al.* (2018) Improved EGFR mutation detection using combined exosomal RNA and circulating tumor DNA in NSCLC patient plasma. *Ann Oncol* **29**: 700–706.

25. Castillo J, Bernard V, San Lucas FA, *et al.* (2017) Surfaceome profiling enables isolation of cancer-specific exosomal cargo in liquid biopsies from pancreatic cancer patients. *Ann Oncol* **29**: 223–239.

26. Peinado H, Zhang H, Matei IR, *et al.* (2017) Pre-metastatic niches: organ-specific homes for metastases. *Nat Rev Cancer* **17**: 302–317.

27. Xu J-Y, Chen G-H, Yang Y-J. (2017) Exosomes: a rising star in falling hearts. *Front Physiol* **8**: 494.

28. Baglio SR, Pegtel DM, Baldini N. (2012) Mesenchymal stem cell secreted vesicles provide novel opportunities in (stem) cell-free therapy. *Front Physiol* **3**: 359.

29. Ailawadi S, Wang X, Gu H, Fan G-C. (2015) Pathologic function and therapeutic potential of exosomes in cardiovascular disease. *Biochim Biophys Acta* **1852**: 1–11.

30. Lai RC, Arslan F, Lee MM, *et al.* (2010) Exosome secreted by MSC reduces myocardial ischemia/reperfusion injury. *Stem Cell Res* **4**: 214–222.

31. Saman S, Kim W, Raya M, *et al.* (2012) Exosome-associated tau is secreted in tauopathy models and is selectively phosphorylated in cerebrospinal fluid in early Alzheimer disease. *J Biol Chem* **287**: 3842–3849.

32. Fais S, O'Driscoll L, Borras FE, *et al.* (2016) Evidence-based clinical use of Nanoscale extracellular vesicles in *Nanomedicine* **10**: 3886–3899.

33. van Niel G, D'Angelo G, Raposo G. (2018) Shedding light on the cell biology of extracellular vesicles. *Nat Rev Mol Cell Biol* **19**: 213–228.

34. Stoorvogel W. (2015) Resolving sorting mechanisms into exosomes. *Cell Res* **25**: 531–532.

35. Möbius W, Ohno-Iwashita Y, van Donselaar EG, *et al.* (2002) Immuno-electron microscopic localization of cholesterol using biotinylated and non-cytolytic perfringolysin O. *J Histochem Cytochem* **50**: 43–55.

36. Wollert T, Wunder C, Lippincott-Schwartz J, Hurley JH. (2009) Membrane scission by the ESCRT-III complex. *Nature* **458**: 172–177.

37. Stuffers S, Wegner CS, Stenmark H, Brech A. (2009) Multivesicular endosome biogenesis in the absence of ESCRTs. *Traffic* **10**: 925–937.

38. Colombo M, Moita C, van Niel G, *et al*. (2013) Analysis of ESCRT functions in exosome biogenesis, composition and secretion highlights the heterogeneity of extracellular vesicles. *J Cell Sci* **126**: 5553–5565.

39. Hurley JH, Hanson PI. (2010) Membrane budding and scission by the ESCRT machinery: it's all in the neck. *Nat Rev Mol Cell Biol* **11**: 556–566.

40. Christ L, Raiborg C, Wenzel EM, Campsteijn C, Stenmark H. (2017) Cellular functions and molecular mechanisms of the ESCRT membrane-scission machinery. *Trends Biochem Sci* **42**: 42–56.

41. Baietti MF, Zhang Z, Mortier E, *et al*. (2012) Syndecan-syntenin-ALIX regulates the biogenesis of exosomes. *Nat Cell Biol* **14**: 677–685.

42. Villarroya-Beltri C, Baixauli F, Gutiérrez-Vázquez C, Sánchez-Madrid F, Mittelbrunn M. (2014) Sorting it out: regulation of exosome loading. *Semin Cancer Biol* **28**: 3–13.

43. Trajkovic K, Hsu C, Chiantia S, *et al*. (2008) Ceramide triggers budding of exosome vesicles into multivesicular endosomes. *Science* **319**: 1244–1247.

44. van Niel G, Charrin S, Simoes S, *et al*. (2011) The tetraspanin CD63 regulates ESCRT-independent and -dependent Endosomal sorting during melanogenesis. *Dev Cell* **21**: 708–721.

45. Geminard C, de Gassart A, Blanc L, Vidal M. (2004) Degradation of AP2 during reticulocyte maturation enhances binding of hsc70 and Alix to a common site on TFR for sorting into exosomes. *Traffic* **5**: 181–193.

46. de Gassart A, Geminard C, Fevrier B, Raposo G, Vidal M. (2003) Lipid raft-associated protein sorting in exosomes. *Blood* **102**: 4336–4344.

47. Colombo M, Raposo G, Thery C. (2014) Biogenesis, secretion, and intercellular interactions of exosomes and other extracellular vesicles. *Annu Rev Cell Dev Biol* **30**: 255–289.

48. Haraszti RA, Didiot M-C, Sapp E, *et al*. (2016) High-resolution proteomic and lipidomic analysis of exosomes and microvesicles from different cell sources. *J Extracell Vesicles* **5**: 32570.

49. Jenjaroenpun P, Kremenska Y, Nair VM, Kremenskoy M, Joseph B, Kurochkin IV. (2013) Characterization of RNA in exosomes secreted by human breast cancer cell lines using next-generation sequencing. *PeerJ* **1**: e201.

50. Wang K, Zhang S, Weber J, Baxter D, Galas DJ. (2010) Export of microRNAs and microRNA-protective protein by mammalian cells. *Nucleic Acids Res* **38**: 7248–7259.

51. Li L, Li C, Wang S, *et al.* (2016) Exosomes derived from hypoxic oral squamous cell carcinoma cells deliver miR-21 to normoxic cells to elicit a prometastatic phenotype. *Cancer Res* **76**: 1770–1780.

52. Ramakrishnaiah V, Thumann C, Fofana I, *et al.* (2013) Exosome-mediated transmission of hepatitis C virus between human hepatoma Huh7.5 cells. *Proc Natl Acad Sci USA* **110**: 13109–13113.

53. Fong MY, Zhou W, Liu L, *et al.* (2015) Breast-cancer-secreted miR-122 reprograms glucose metabolism in premetastatic niche to promote metastasis. *Nat Cell Biol* **17**: 183–194.

54. Ben-Dov IZ, Whalen VM, Goilav B, Max KEA, Tuschl T. (2016) Cell and Microvesicle urine microRNA deep sequencing profiles from healthy individuals: observations with potential impact on biomarker studies. *PLoS ONE* **11**: e0147249.

55. Batagov AO, Kurochkin IV. (2013) Exosomes secreted by human cells transport largely mRNA fragments that are enriched in the 3′-untranslated regions. *Biol Direct* **8**: 12.

56. San Lucas FA, Allenson K, Bernard V, *et al.* (2015) Minimally invasive genomic and transcriptomic profiling of visceral cancers by next-generation sequencing of circulating exosomes. *Ann Oncol* **27**(4): 635–641.

57. Kahlert C, Melo SA, Melo SA, *et al.* (2014) Identification of double-stranded genomic DNA spanning all chromosomes with mutated KRAS and p53 DNA in the serum exosomes of patients with pancreatic cancer. *J Biol Chem* **289**: 3869–3875.

58. Mittelbrunn M, Gutiérrez-Vázquez C, Villarroya-Beltri C, *et al.* (2011) Unidirectional transfer of microRNA-loaded exosomes from T cells to antigen-presenting cells. *Nat Commun* **2**: 282.

59. Mateescu B, Kowal EJK, van Balkom BWM, *et al.* (2017) Obstacles and opportunities in the functional analysis of extracellular vesicle RNA-an ISEV position paper. *J Extracell Vesicles* **6**: 1286095.

60. Villarroya-Beltri C, Gutiérrez-Vázquez C, Sánchez-Cabo F, *et al.* (2013) Sumoylated hnRNPA2B1 controls the sorting of miRNAs into exosomes through binding to specific motifs. *Nat Commun* **4**: 2980.

61. Koppers-Lalic D, Hackenberg M, Bijnsdorp IV, *et al.* (2014) Nontemplated nucleotide additions distinguish the small RNA composition in cells from exosomes. *Cell Rep* **8**: 1649–1658.

62. Gibbings DJ, Ciaudo C, Erhardt M, Voinnet O. (2009) Multivesicular bodies associate with components of miRNA effector complexes and modulate miRNA activity. *Nat Cell Biol* **11**: 1143–1149.

63. Kosaka N, Iguchi H, Yoshioka Y, Takeshita F, Matsuki Y, Ochiya T. (2010) Secretory mechanisms and intercellular transfer of microRNAs in living cells. *J Biol Chem* **285**: 17442–17452.

64. Squadrito ML, Baer C, Burdet F, *et al.* (2014) Endogenous RNAs modulate microRNA sorting to exosomes and transfer to acceptor cells. *Cell Rep* **8**: 1432–1446.

65. Cheng L, Sharples RA, Scicluna BJ, Hill AF. (2014) Exosomes provide a protective and enriched source of miRNA for biomarker profiling compared to intracellular and cell-free blood. *J Extracell Vesicles* **3**: 23743.

66. Shelke GV, Lasser C, Gho YS, Lotvall J. (2014) Importance of exosome depletion protocols to eliminate functional and RNA-containing extracellular vesicles from fetal bovine serum. *J Extracell Vesicles* **3**: 24783.

67. Tang Y-T, Huang Y-Y, Zheng L, *et al.* (2017) Comparison of isolation methods of exosomes and exosomal RNA from cell culture medium and serum. *Int J Mol Med* **40**: 834–844.

68. Becker C, Hammerle-Fickinger A, Riedmaier I, Pfaffl MW. (2010) mRNA and microRNA quality control for RT-qPCR analysis. *Methods* **50**: 237–243.

69. Aranda R, Dineen SM, Craig RL, Guerrieri RA, Robertson JM. (2009) Comparison and evaluation of RNA quantification methods using viral, prokaryotic, and eukaryotic RNA over a 10(4) concentration range. *Anal Biochem* **387**: 122–127.

70. Kim Y-K, Yeo J, Kim B, Ha M, Kim VN. (2012) Short structured RNAs with low GC content are selectively lost during extraction from a small number of cells. *Mol Cell* **46**: 893–895.

71. Huang X, Yuan T, Tschannen M, *et al.* (2013) Characterization of human plasma-derived exosomal RNAs by deep sequencing. *BMC Genomics* **14**: 319.

72. Hill AF, Pegtel DM, Lambertz U, *et al.* (2013) ISEV position paper: extracellular vesicle RNA analysis and bioinformatics. *J Extracell Vesicles* **2**: 22859.

73. Iwakawa H-O, Tomari Y. (2015) The functions of MicroRNAs: mRNA decay and translational repression. *Trends Cell Biol.* **25**: 651–665.

74. Bhome R, Del Vecchio F, Lee G-H, *et al.* (2018) Exosomal microRNAs (exomiRs): small molecules with a big role in cancer. *Cancer Lett* **420**: 228–235.

75. Lotvall J, Hill AF, Hochberg F, *et al.* (2014) Minimal experimental requirements for definition of extracellular vesicles and their functions: a position statement from the International Society for Extracellular Vesicles. *J Extracell Vesicles* **3**: 26913.

76. Cointe S, Judicone C, Robert S, *et al.* (2017) Standardization of microparticle enumeration across different flow cytometry platforms: results of a multicenter collaborative workshop. *J Thromb Haemost* **15**: 187–193.

77. van der Pol E, Hoekstra AG, Sturk A, Otto C, van Leeuwen TG, Nieuwland R. (2010) Optical and non-optical methods for detection and characterization of microparticles and exosomes. *J Thromb Haemost* **8**: 2596–2607.

78. Dragovic RA, Gardiner C, Brooks AS, *et al.* (2011) Sizing and phenotyping of cellular vesicles using nanoparticle tracking analysis. *Nanomedicine* **7**: 780–788.

79. Soo CY, Song Y, Zheng Y, *et al.* (2012) Nanoparticle tracking analysis monitors microvesicle and exosome secretion from immune cells. *Immunology* **136**: 192–197.

80. van der Pol E, Coumans FAW, Sturk A, Nieuwland R, van Leeuwen TG. (2014) Refractive index determination of nanoparticles in suspension using nanoparticle tracking analysis. *Nano Lett* **14**: 6195–6201.

81. Vogel R, Coumans FAW, Maltesen RG, *et al.* (2016) A standardized method to determine the concentration of extracellular vesicles using tunable resistive pulse sensing. *J Extracell Vesicles* **5**: 31242.

82. Smith ZJ, Lee C, Rojalin T, *et al.* (2015) Single exosome study reveals subpopulations distributed among cell lines with variability related to membrane content. *J Extracell Vesicles* **4**: 28533.

83. Crescitelli R, Lasser C, Szabó TG, *et al.* (2013) Distinct RNA profiles in subpopulations of extracellular vesicles: apoptotic bodies, microvesicles and exosomes. *J Extracell Vesicles* **2**: 20677.

84. Raiborg C, Stenmark H. (2009) The ESCRT machinery in endosomal sorting of ubiquitylated membrane proteins. *Nature* **458**: 445–452.

85. Xu R, Greening DW, Rai A, Ji H, Simpson RJ. (2015) Highly-purified exosomes and shed microvesicles isolated from the human colon cancer cell line LIM1863 by sequential centrifugal ultrafiltration are biochemically and functionally distinct. *Methods* **87**: 11–25.

86. Aatonen MT, Ohman T, Nyman TA, Laitinen S, Grönholm M, Siljander PRM. (2014) Isolation and characterization of platelet-derived extracellular vesicles. *J Extracell Vesicles* **3**: 24692.

87. Oksvold MP, Kullmann A, Forfang L, *et al.* (2014) Expression of B-cell surface antigens in subpopulations of exosomes released from B-cell lymphoma cells. *Clin Ther* **36**: 847–862.e1.

88. Yoshioka Y, Konishi Y, Kosaka N, Katsuda T, Kato T, Ochiya T. (2013) Comparative marker analysis of extracellular vesicles in different human cancer types. *J Extracell Vesicles* **2**: 20424.

89. Kim D-K, Nishida H, An SY, Shetty AK, Bartosh TJ, Prockop DJ. (2016) Chromatographically isolated CD63+CD81+ extracellular vesicles from mesenchymal stromal cells rescue cognitive impairments after TBI. *Proc Natl Acad Sci USA* **113**: 170–175.

90. Belov L, Matic KJ, Hallal S, Best OG, Mulligan SP, Christopherson RI. (2016) Extensive surface protein profiles of extracellular vesicles from cancer cells may provide diagnostic signatures from blood samples. *J Extracell Vesicles* **5**: 25355.

91. Samsonov R, Shtam T, Burdakov V, *et al.* (2016) Lectin-induced agglutination method of urinary exosomes isolation followed by mi-RNA analysis: application for prostate cancer diagnostic. *Prostate* **76**: 68–79.

92. Wei Z, Batagov AO, Carter DRF, Krichevsky AM. (2016) Fetal bovine serum RNA interferes with the cell culture derived extracellular RNA. *Sci Rep* **6**: 31175.

93. Witwer KW, Buzás EI, Bemis LT, *et al.* (2013) Standardization of sample collection, isolation and analysis methods in extracellular vesicle research. *J Extracell Vesicles* **2**. doi: 10.3402/jev.v2i0.20360. eCollection 2013

94. Lacroix R, Judicone C, Mooberry M, *et al.* (2013) Standardization of pre-analytical variables in plasma microparticle determination: results of the international society on thrombosis and Haemostasis SSC collaborative workshop. *J Thromb Haemost* **11**: 1190–1193.

95. Beutler E, Gelbart T, Kuhl W. (1990) Interference of heparin with the polymerase chain reaction. *BioTechniques* **9**: 166.

96. Lippi G, Salvagno GL, Montagnana M, Franchini M, Guidi GC. (2006) Venous stasis and routine hematologic testing. *Clin Lab Haematol* **28**: 332–337.

97. Hefler L, Grimm C, Leodolter S, Tempfer C. (2004) To butterfly or to needle: the pilot phase. *Ann Intern Med* **140**: 935–936.

98. Gyorgy B, Pálóczi K, Kovács A, *et al.* (2014) Improved circulating micro-particle analysis in acid-citrate dextrose (ACD) anticoagulant tube. *Thromb Res* **133**: 285–292.

99. Lacroix R, Judicone C, Poncelet P, *et al.* (2012) Impact of pre-analytical parameters on the measurement of circulating microparticles: towards standardization of protocol. *J Thromb Haemost* **10**: 437–446.

100. Coumans FAW, Brisson AR, Buzas EI, *et al.* (2017) Methodological guide-lines to study extracellular vesicles. *Circ Res* **120**: 1632–1648.

101. Maroto R, Zhao Y, Jamaluddin M, *et al.* (2017) Effects of storage tempera-ture on airway exosome integrity for diagnostic and functional analyses. *J Extracell Vesicles* **6**: 1359478.

102. Trummer A, De Rop C, Tiede A, Ganser A, Eisert R. (2009) Recovery and composition of microparticles after snap-freezing depends on thawing temperature. *Blood Coagul Fibrinolysis* **20**: 52–56.

103. Zarovni N, Corrado A, Guazzi P, *et al.* (2015) Integrated isolation and quantitative analysis of exosome shuttled proteins and nucleic acids using immunocapture approaches. *Methods* **87**: 46–58.

104. Cvjetkovic A, Lotvall J, Lasser C. (2014) The influence of rotor type and centrifugation time on the yield and purity of extracellular vesicles. *J Extracell Vesicles* **3**: 23111.

105. Chevillet JR, Kang Q, Ruf IK, *et al.* (2014) Quantitative and stoichiometric analysis of the microRNA content of exosomes. *Proc Natl Acad Sci USA* **111**: 14888–14893.

106. Grapp M, Wrede A, Schweizer M, *et al.* (2013) Choroid plexus transcytosis and exosome shuttling deliver folate into brain parenchyma. *Nat Commun* **4**: 2123.

107. Miranda KC, Bond DT, Levin JZ, *et al.* (2014) Massively parallel sequencing of human urinary exosome/microvesicle RNA reveals a predominance of non-coding RNA. *PLoS ONE* **9**: e96094.

108. Cheruvanky A, Zhou H, Pisitkun T, *et al*. (2007) Rapid isolation of urinary exosomal biomarkers using a nanomembrane ultrafiltration concentrator. *Am J Physiol Renal Physiol* **292**: F1657–F1661.

109. Liga A, Vliegenthart ADB, Oosthuyzen W, Dear JW, Kersaudy-Kerhoas M. (2015) Exosome isolation: a microfluidic road-map. *Lab Chip* **15**: 2388–2394.

110. Rider MA, Hurwitz SN, Meckes DG. (2016) ExtraPEG: a polyethylene glycol-based method for enrichment of extracellular vesicles. *Sci Rep* **6**: 23978.

111. Gyorgy B, Módos K, Pállinger E, *et al*. (2011) Detection and isolation of cell-derived microparticles are compromised by protein complexes resulting from shared biophysical parameters. *Blood* **117**: e39–e48.

112. Zhao Z, Yang Y, Zeng Y, He M. (2016) A microfluidic ExoSearch chip for multiplexed exosome detection towards blood-based ovarian cancer diagnosis. *Lab Chip* **16**: 489–496.

113. Kanwar SS, Dunlay CJ, Simeone DM, Nagrath S. (2014) Microfluidic device (ExoChip) for on-chip isolation, quantification and characterization of circulating exosomes. *Lab Chip* **14**: 1891–900.

114. Kang D, Oh S, Ahn S-M, Lee B-H, Moon MH. (2008) Proteomic analysis of exosomes from human neural stem cells by flow field-flow fractionation and nanoflow liquid chromatography-tandem mass spectrometry. *J Proteome Res* **7**: 3475–3480.

115. Lee K, Shao H, Weissleder R, Lee H. (2015) Acoustic purification of extracellular microvesicles. *ACS Nano* **9**: 2321–2327.

116. Ding M, Wang C, Lu X, *et al*. (2018) Comparison of commercial exosome isolation kits for circulating exosomal microRNA profiling. *Anal Bioanal Chem* **410**: 3805–3814.

117. Helwa I, Cai J, Drewry MD, *et al*. (2017) A comparative study of serum exosome isolation using differential ultracentrifugation and three commercial reagents. *PLoS ONE* **12**: e0170628.

118. EV-TRACK Consortium, Van Deun J, Mestdagh P, *et al*. (2017) EV-TRACK: transparent reporting and centralizing knowledge in extracellular vesicle research. *Nat Methods* **14**: 228–232.

119. Van Deun J, Mestdagh P, Sormunen R, *et al*. (2014) The impact of disparate isolation methods for extracellular vesicles on downstream RNA profiling. *J Extracell Vesicles* **3**: 24858.

120. Andreu Z, Rivas E, Sanguino-Pascual A, *et al.* (2016) Comparative analysis of EV isolation procedures for miRNAs detection in serum samples. *J Extracell Vesicles* **5**: 31655.

121. Nakai W, Yoshida T, Diez D, *et al.* (2016) A novel affinity-based method for the isolation of highly purified extracellular vesicles. *Sci Rep* **6**: 33935.

122. Tauro BJ, Greening DW, Mathias RA, *et al.* (2012) Comparison of ultra-centrifugation, density gradient separation, and immunoaffinity capture methods for isolating human colon cancer cell line LIM1863-derived exosomes. *Methods* **56**: 293–304.

123. Arraud N, Linares R, Tan S, *et al.* (2014) Extracellular vesicles from blood plasma: determination of their morphology, size, phenotype and concentration. *J Thromb Haemost* **12**: 614–627.

124. Groot Kormelink T, Arkesteijn GJA, Nauwelaers FA, van den Engh G, Nolte-'t Hoen ENM, Wauben MHM. (2016) Prerequisites for the analysis and sorting of extracellular vesicle subpopulations by high-resolution flow cytometry. *Cytometry A* **89**: 135–147.

125. Arroyo JD, Chevillet JR, Kroh EM, *et al.* (2011) Argonaute2 complexes carry a population of circulating microRNAs independent of vesicles in human plasma. *Proc Natl Acad Sci USA* **108**: 5003–5008.

126. Vickers KC, Palmisano BT, Shoucri BM, Shamburek RD, Remaley AT. (2011) MicroRNAs are transported in plasma and delivered to recipient cells by high-density lipoproteins. *Nat Cell Biol* **13**: 423–433.

127. Sódar BW, Kittel A, Pálóczi K, *et al.* (2016) Low-density lipoprotein mimics blood plasma-derived exosomes and microvesicles during isolation and detection. *Sci Rep* **6**: 24316.

Chapter 9

DNA Methylation Analysis of Circulating DNA Biomarkers

Kristina Warton, Clare Stirzaker, Goli Samimi and Susan Clark

Abstract

DNA methylation alterations are often more consistent between individual tumors than mutations, and offer an alternative target for circulating DNA assays in cancer. Here we summarize different approaches to methylation analysis, with a focus on their technical parameters in the context of circulating DNA research.

DNA Methylation

DNA methylation is the presence of a methyl group covalently linked to the cytosine base in the context of a CpG dinucleotide (CpG site)[1] and provides a layer of epigenetic information specifying how the DNA sequence may be interpreted in the context of individual cell and tissue biology.[2] Approximately 70% of gene promoters are associated with regions that have maintained CpG sites through evolution, known as CpG islands.[3] Generally, unmethylated CpG island–associated promoters are more loosely packaged and therefore accessible to transcription factors, such that the gene can be activated in response to the appropriate stimuli. In contrast, methylated CpG island promoters are commonly more densely packaged and as such prevent accessibility to transcription factor binding and corresponding gene activation. DNA methylation patterns are established during cell differentiation and vary by cell type,[4] and this epigenetic variation allows signalling pathways to elicit different transcriptional responses depending on the tissue and cell type involved. Cell-type DNA methylation patterns are preserved when DNA is released from necrotic or apoptotic cells into the circulating cell-free DNA (cirDNA) pool and is thus a ready source of biomarkers accessible via a "liquid biopsy" blood draw. In this chapter, we describe different methods for analyzing methylation of cirDNA at candidate regions that may have biomarker potential and highlight the technical considerations when assays are applied to cirDNA samples.

cirDNA Methylation as a Cell-of-Origin Biomarker

Since DNA methylation is involved in cell differentiation, individual cell types defining a tissue carry distinct methylation footprints.[5-7] For this reason, the different cell types contributing to the cirDNA pool can be identified by the methylation pattern detected in the cirDNA. DNA methylation analysis from blood samples has shown that the bulk of cirDNA in healthy individuals is derived from leukocytes, erythrocyte progenitors, and endothelial cells, with a minor contribution from hepatocytes.[8-11] Tissues compromised by pathological processes experience higher cell death, with the appearance of corresponding cell-specific DNA methylation pattern in plasma. For example, patients with recently diagnosed diabetes show an increase in pancreatic β-cell cirDNA,[12] while hepatocyte cirDNA is increased in patients experiencing rejection of a liver transplant and sepsis.[13]

cirDNA Methylation as a Cancer Biomarker

Aberrant DNA methylation patterns are a frequent event associated with carcinogenesis and commonly occur early in the tumor cell formation process.[5,14] Promoter CpG island methylation is one of the mechanisms by which tumor suppressor genes are inactivated, leading to uncontrolled cell division.[15] Alterations in DNA methylation patterns in gene promoters and intergenic regions are also associated with different characteristics of the tumor, including histological and molecular subtypes that can shape the signalling pathways involved in tumorigenesis.[16] Cancer-related DNA methylation changes are also commonly shared within a given type of tumor. For example, the *HOXA9* promoter and the *EN1* promoter are methylated in 95% and 80% of high-grade serous ovarian tumors, respectively, and unmethylated in healthy ovarian epithelium,[17] while the *14-3-3 sigma* promoter is methylated in 96% of breast tumors, and unmethylated in healthy breast tissue.[18] Methylation-specific PCR assays that detect the methylation status of a given promoter are routinely applied to cohorts of tissue samples.[19] A positive outcome of the PCR is indicative of DNA methylation, with no DNA sequencing required.

Detection of circulating tumor–derived DNA (ctDNA) in blood plasma through tumor-specific methylation patterns also offers an alternative or complementary approach to the detection of cancer-derived genetic mutations.[20] For example, the two genes most commonly mutated in breast cancer, *TP53* and *PK3KCA*, are only altered in 37% and 36% of cases, respectively.[21] Even when a cancer is characterized by mutations in a particular gene, as is the case with *TP53* in ovarian cancer,[22,23] those mutations are typically spread over many thousands of base pairs of DNA. Frequent, consistent point mutations, such as those in *KRAS* in pancreatic cancer,[20] are the exception rather than the norm. This diversity provides a challenge for the design of targeted assays to detect ctDNA in blood. Prior knowledge of specific mutations, obtained from sequencing tumor tissue DNA, is a straightforward and effective approach but requires labor-intensive characterization of each individual patient tumor before the ctDNA assay can be created[24]; it is therefore not a strategy applicable in the context of cancer diagnostic tests. In cancer types that have a degree of consistency in their mutations, DNA sequencing panels targeting the regions of interest can be applied directly to cirDNA.[25]

Analysis of DNA Methylation

A wide range of techniques have been developed for the study of DNA methylation. While most of these approaches incorporate a bisulfite treatment step,[19,26,27] enzymatic cytosine conversion is also possible[28] and several approaches are bisulfite free.[29,30] These protocols have been largely developed for the analysis of relatively abundant, high–molecular weight (HMW) genomic DNA, and are now being translated with varying success to ctDNA analysis. In contrast to genomic DNA, ctDNA is typically found at low concentrations and is heavily fragmented. Here, we review the different methods of cirDNA methylation analysis and consider their advantages and limitations in the context of investigating cirDNA.

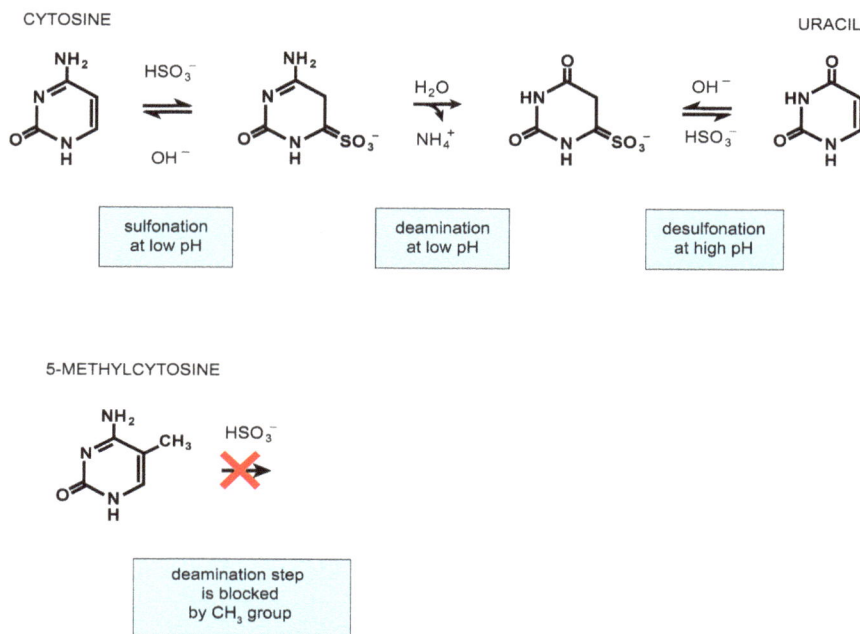

Fig. 1: Conversion of unmethylated cytosines to uracil by bisulfite treatment. Methylated cytosine does not undergo the reaction as the deamination step is blocked by the methyl group.

Bisulfite-Based Methods

Bisulfite conversion of DNA has been the backbone of DNA methylation analysis for over three decades.[31–33] Bisulfite reacts with unmethylated cytosine by nucleophilic attack of the C6 carbon, and the sulfonate group can then be removed via hydrolytic deamination with alkali treatment to produce uracil (Fig. 1). Methylated cytosine does not undergo this reaction to an appreciable extent and remains unchanged. Hence following bisulfite treatment, all unmethylated cytosines are converted to uracil, while methylated cytosines remain as cytosine, resulting in sequence differences between methylated and unmethylated DNA (Fig. 2). The methylation sites can then be analyzed by PCR and sequencing.

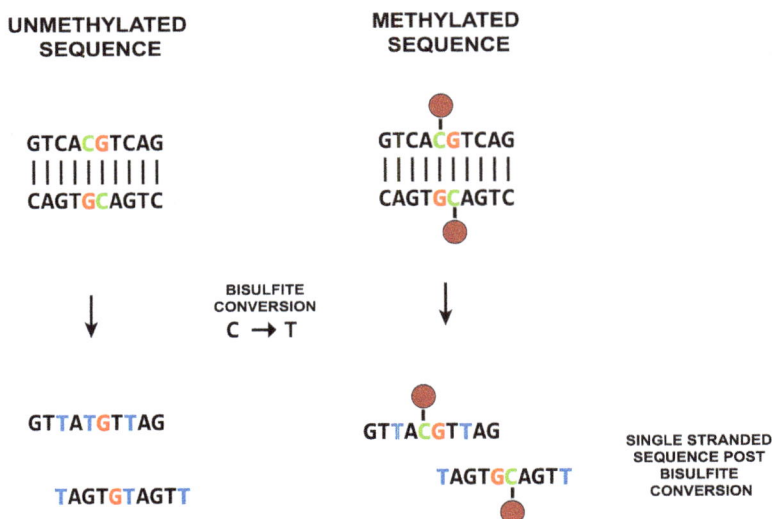

Fig. 2:   Bisulfite treatment creates a sequence difference between methylated and unmethylated DNA after conversion of unmethylated cytosines to uracil.

A large number of bisulfite conversion kits are commercially available; however, relatively few studies have evaluated these specifically in the context of cirDNA.[34–37] Techniques that bisulfite convert cirDNA face the same challenges as techniques that purify cirDNA, namely, that the target DNA is in low abundance and fragmented. However, one advantage of cirDNA is that it undergoes less fragmentation than HMW genomic DNA during bisulfite treatment, as the short fragments are resistant to further degradation.[38,39]

As short DNA fragments do not have the same matrix binding and recovery characteristics as large DNA fragments (see Chapter 4), for the purpose of cirDNA studies it is important that methods are evaluated using DNA input of the appropriate size. For example, Worm Orntoft and colleagues used a 131-bp custom PCR product to evaluate the performance of 11 commercial bisulfite conversion kits and one in-house method.[36] They observed a large variability in kit performance, which was more pronounced for the small (131 bp) PCR product than large genomic leukocyte DNA. The EZ Methylation-Direct kit from Zymo Research was the highest rated kit, with the Epijet kit from ThermoFisher Scientific a close second. Holmes and colleagues compared nine different bisulfite conversion kits, manufactured by three different biotech companies[34]; however, this study only used FFPE DNA, also a fragmented substrate, in the direct kit comparisons. The kits that were selected all performed with similar efficiency; however, a decrease in the recovery of FFPE bisulfite-treated DNA compared to tissue DNA was reported.[34] Only one kit, the innuConvert Bisulphite Body Fluids Kit, was tested for performance with plasma cirDNA samples and yielded ~150 ng cirDNA per mL of plasma. This unexpectedly high yield may be due to leukocyte lysis during pre-processing blood storage (Chapter 2), as sample blood sample handling parameters are not reported in the study. Finally, a study used qPCR to compare recovery of cirDNA that was bisulfite converted using either the EpiTect or the EpiTect Fast kits from Qiagen and found that the EpiTect Fast resulted in approximately double the yield as well as allowing more rapid sample processing.[38]

PCR of Bisulfite-Converted cirDNA

Following bisulfite conversion, DNA can be selectively amplified and quantitated by PCR. Bisulfite-treated DNA templates are generally more challenging to amplify; as in the initial PCR cycles, the DNA polymerase must contend with uracil instead of thymine in the DNA backbone,[40] and runs of consecutive dTs are more frequent following the conversion of unmethylated cytosines.[41]

In the following, we address considerations for PCR of bisulfite-converted cirDNA. Despite these challenges, PCR is commonly used to analyze DNA methylation in tissue and cirDNA; indeed, a PCR assay for the methylated *SEPT9* promoter in cirDNA forms the basis of an FDA-approved blood test for colorectal cancer.[42] Blood plasma tests for methylated cirDNA biomarkers for hepatocellular carcinoma and lung cancer are also regulatory agency approved (reviewed by Ref. (19)).[19]

(i) Amplicon size

Amplicon size is an important consideration in any cirDNA PCR design (Chapter 5) but even more so for bisulfite-treated DNA and cirDNA. cirDNA occurs mainly as fragments ~167 bp in size, hence PCR assays targeting sequences above this size will have limited available DNA template. Below 167 bp, assay sensitivity progressively increases with decreasing amplicon size, reflecting a higher number of available intact targets.[43] Bisulfite treatment leads to fragmentation and loss of template[44]; hence small amplicons are important for maximizing available target sequence; however, a recent study has shown that cirDNA has some resistance to fragmentation during bisulfite treatment, most likely due to its shorter length.[38] There is a lower limit to PCR product size, which must accommodate the length of both primers, and often a probe sequence. Where the PCR product is to be analyzed by gel electrophoresis, the size of the product must be distinguishable from the size of any potential primer dimer.

(ii) Effect of nucleosome positioning

Regions of differential methylation that regulate gene expression are typically found in CpG islands associated with gene promoters.[45] Nucleosomes at the start sites of active genes are not randomly distributed; rather, they are regularly and consistently positioned with a nucleosome-free region at the transcription start site (TSS).[46] Indeed, the cirDNA fragmentation pattern at TSS sites has allowed researchers to determine whether a particular gene is active in the cells that contributed to the cirDNA pool and the identification of the cells of origin.[46]

Due to the regular nucleosome spacing at TSS sites, care must be taken when designing methylation-specific primers (MSP) at gene promoters. If the PCR assay spans the TSS of an active gene, a negative result may not reflect the methylation status of the gene but rather the fact the DNA is cleaved at the TSS and thus not available as a template for PCR. For example, before the fragmentation pattern of cirDNA (that stems from the regular spacing of nucleosomes at TSS sites) had been described in the literature, Jahr and colleagues designed a PCR assay to test whether endothelial cells contributed DNA to the cirDNA pool.[47] This assay targeted the unmethylated *E-selectin* promoter, known to be expressed specifically in endothelial cells.[48] The assay successfully amplified genomic endothelial cell DNA but generated no PCR product when cirDNA was used as the template, leading to the conclusion that endothelial cell DNA was not present in the cirDNA pool. However, this negative result was artifactual, and due to the primers spanning the TSS. Fifteen years later, Moss and colleagues used Illumina methylation array data to show that endothelial cells contributed approximately 10% of the total cirDNA in healthy individuals.[8]

(iii) Primer design

Methylation-specific PCR: Depending on the needs of the assay, PCR of bisulfite-converted DNA can be designed to specifically amplify either the methylated (MSP) or unmethylated sequence (USP), or amplify both unmethylated and methylated sequences nonselectively. Methylation-specific PCR is dependent on mismatches where the primers overlap CpG sites. In theory, and occasionally in practice,[49] a single CpG site resulting in a primer-template mismatch is sufficient to make the primers specific for a selected methylation state, but this is dependent on individual sequence characteristics such as annealing temperature bias. In general, at least three mismatches, at CpG sites, between each of the primers and the undesired template provide a sufficient basis for developing a specific PCR reaction, but once again, this is dependent on individual sequence. A critical consideration is the positioning of the mismatches within the primer, with mismatches within the 3′-most bases providing the highest specificity.[49,50]

Unbiased PCR: Unbiased PCR, that is PCR amplifying both the methylated and the unmethylated target with equal efficiency, is carried out when the relative proportions of the methylated and unmethylated region are to be determined by a downstream technique, such as next-generation sequencing or clonal sequencing. Equal amplification of both targets is difficult as the base pair composition post-bisulfite treatment is very different. While the primers may be designed to be unbiased, PCR bias can occur due to the inherent difference in sequence of methylated and unmethylated strands.[51] PCR conditions need to be optimized and primers ideally are designed such that they do not span sequences containing CpG sites or have an inosine residue to pair with the C of the CpG site.[52]

In methylation analysis, the DNA molecules of interest can occur in a background excess of opposite methylation status DNA. This is particularly the case when detecting methylated tumor DNA in plasma or DNA contributions from rare cell types. In this scenario, the PCR reaction needs to not only efficiently amplify the desired target but also avoid the opposite methylation status DNA, which has a very similar sequence. DNA duplex stability decreases with increasing temperature and decreasing magnesium, so the unspecific PCR reaction with the primer mismatch can be made less efficient, or eliminated by raising annealing temperature or lowering magnesium. However, this can also decrease the efficiency of the perfectly matched primer reaction, so developing methylation-specific PCR assays involves systematically identifying temperature/magnesium combinations at which priming of the nonspecific target does not occur while retaining sufficient reaction efficiency for the specific target. Selected PCR additives can also be empirically tested for their effect on the specificity and efficiency of the reaction, with dimethyl sulfoxide having proved useful for aiding the amplification of GC-rich templates.[53]

"Alternate" strand PCR assay design: Following bisulfite treatment, there are two distinct DNA sequences available for assays testing the methylation status of a region of interest. In an unmethylated C–G pair, only the C is modified by bisulfite treatment, while the G remains unchanged, forming at T–G mismatch. Thus the two DNA strands are no longer complementary and offer two different targets, each of which can be used to determine the methylation status of the original (Fig. 3). In cases where one DNA strand is not amenable to PCR, either because a PCR assay with a suitable annealing temperature and favorable self-complementarity parameters cannot be designed, or because the PCR can be designed but fails in laboratory testing, it is well worth attempting to design an assay that utilizes the other strand. Thus, each region does offer two options at designing specific and efficient PCRs.

Evaluation of Methylation Following PCR Amplification of Bisulfite-converted cirDNA

(i) Visualizing the PCR product

The PCR product can be visualized by traditional gel electrophoresis or by one of the more recent capillary electrophoresis methods

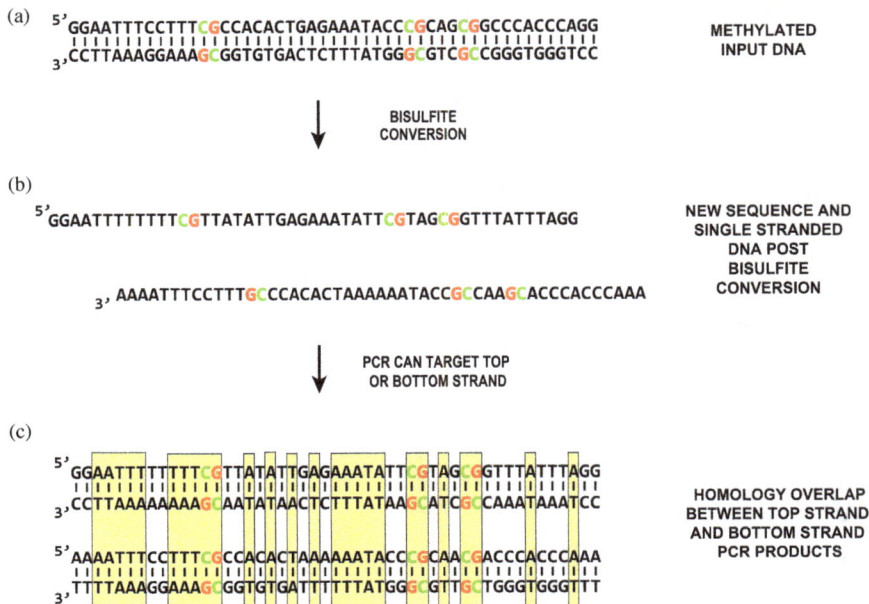

Fig. 3: Following bisulfite conversion, the two DNA strands are no longer complementary.

that also rely on matrix-based DNA separation by size (e.g., Bioanalyzer, TapeStation, Qiaxel, Advanced Analytical Fragment Separator). However, while these methods can determine whether the product is of the expected size, they cannot differentiate between amplification of methylated and unmethylated sequences, as both generate a product of the same length, and additional measures to determine which product was amplified are required.

(ii) Quantitative PCR

Quantitative PCR (qPCR) techniques are equally applicable to bisulfite-treated DNA and bisulfite-untreated DNA. DNA intercalating dyes such as SYTO9 or SYBR Green can be used to quantitate the target of interest, with the additional advantage that the melt curve will vary with the methylation status of the amplified product, thus providing some information regarding the specificity of the reaction. In general, the methylated product will have a higher cytosine content, hence a higher melt temperature; however, this does not apply in cases where differentially methylated cytosines are only found within the primer sequence and not in the region between the primers. This is because every PCR product incorporates primer molecules, and all but the few initial template DNA fragments are copied from primers. Hence, the sequence of a PCR product within the primer regions will always match the primers, even if the product was initially generated by a nonspecific mispriming event. For this reason, only the differentially methylated CpG sites that lie between primers contribute to a melt temperature difference between methylated and unmethylated DNA (Fig. 4).

Methylation-specific qPCR assays that incorporate a probe sequence between the primers (MethylLight) can also be used to quantitate the target template and monitor reaction specificity, as the probe can be designed to overlap CpG sites thereby selectively visualizing amplification of the sequence of interest, and not the related, mismatched DNA. This approach has commonly been used to detect tumor DNA in the cell-free DNA pool.[54,55] Alternately to MethylLight conversion-specific detection of DNA methylation can be achieved using real-time PCR (ConLight-MSP) to avoid false positives that commonly occur in DNA derived from clinical samples.[56]

(iii) Digital PCR

Digital PCR involves partitioning the PCR reaction into tens of thousands of individual reactions and counting how many of these contain amplified product once cycling is finished.[57] Amplified product indicates the presence of a specific target molecule in the

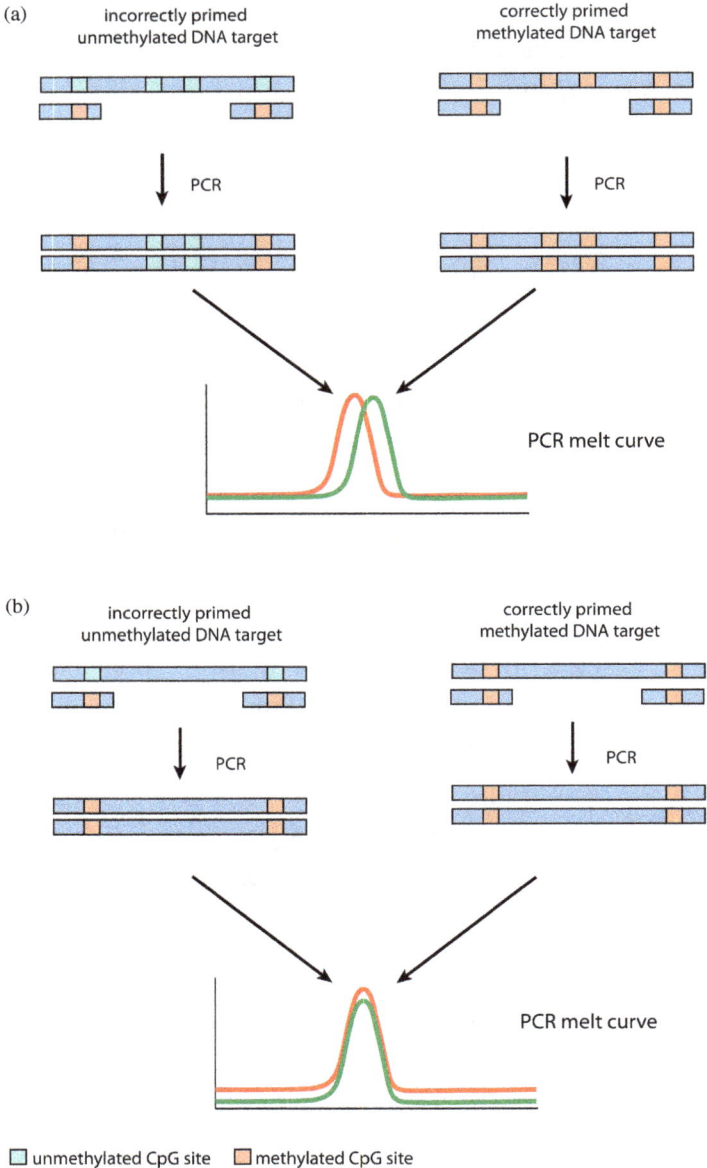

Fig. 4: Mispriming in methylation-specific qPCR (a) When CpG sites with different methylation status are present between the primers, the misprimed product can be distinguished by a different melt temperature. (b) When there are no CpG sites with different methylation status between the primers, the misprimed and the correct PCR product cannot be distinguished by the melt curve.

original mix, so it is effectively counting individual DNA targets. The method does not require a standard curve and provides an increase in sensitivity over traditional qPCR methods. It is particularly suited to cirDNA applications in which low amounts of target template are often a technical hurdle.

An additional benefit of digital PCR relates to the aforementioned difficulty in detecting rare molecules in a high background of DNA with the opposite methylation status. As described, using a probe can selectively visualize amplification of the correct target, but it cannot prevent amplification of the incorrect sequence, which may, if sufficient, decrease the efficiency of the correct reaction, leading to low sensitivity. The partitioning in digital PCR means that in those droplets that contain the correct target, the ratio of correct target to related sequence is much higher; hence inhibition due to related sequence amplification will be less pronounced. In those droplets that contain only the incorrect, related sequence, some amplification may take place, but there will be no fluorescence due to the specificity of the probe.

(iv) Methyl-BEAMing

Methyl-BEAMing (Beads Emulsion Amplification Magnetics) is a digital approach to detect and quantitate DNA methylation in samples, particularly applicable when the methylated molecules are present in a large excess of unmethylated background DNA.[58] The procedure involves methylation-specific amplification of bisulfite-converted DNA in aqueous compartments suspended within an oil phase, which also includes beads that bind amplified PCR product. After amplification is complete, the beads, now coated with selectively amplified DNA, are labelled with hybridization probes and counted by flow cytometry.[58] This method has been used to detect methylated vimentin in plasma from colorectal cancer patients[58] and used to evaluate drug sensitivity in colorectal cancer.[59,60]

Additional Methodologies to Increase the Selectivity of Methylation-Specific PCR

While dye-based and probe-based methods can help determine whether the amplified product is methylated or unmethylated, neither of them contribute to PCR reaction specificity. As described, cirDNA molecules with the methylation status of interest often occur in a background excess of molecules with the opposite methylation status. For a given region of interest, it may only be possible to identify a temperature and magnesium combination in which the amplification of the related sequence is reduced but not eliminated. Additional strategies can then be used to suppress the amplification of the related sequence and create a highly specific PCR assay.

(i) Headloop suppression PCR

The headloop suppression PCR strategy[61] can either be used on its own to selectively amplify DNA with the desired methylation status, or as an adjunct to increase the specificity of MSP.[17] In this method, one or both of the primers contain an additional sequence at the 5′ end, which is complementary to a sequence within the undesired PCR product. In the event that mispriming and DNA extension occurs, the PCR molecule transcribed contains a self-complementary sequence and is able to form a hairpin loop structure that blocks further priming. Because this intramolecular binding is much more efficient than primer annealing, the misprimed sequence is effectively removed from further participating in the PCR reaction. This mechanism is sufficiently efficient that it can give selective amplification even in the absence of methylation-specific sequences within the actual primer, and sensitive down to around 25 pg of target DNA.[61] This method has been successfully used to monitor prostate cancer patients receiving chemotherapy by tracking cirDNA-methylated GSTP1 levels.[62,63]

(ii) HeavyMethyl

Another strategy to prevent the amplification of the unmethylated DNA sequence, known as HeavyMethyl, uses a methylation-specific oligonucleotide blocker.[64] The nonextendable blockers bind within the primer binding sites and prevent the binding of the primers. Together with methylation-specific fluorescent probes, this can be sufficient to selectively amplify methylated DNA even when the primer does not favor the methylated sequence.[64] This approach, together with a MethylLight probe, was successfully used in the SEPT9 assay for the detection of methylated colorectal cancer DNA in patient plasma.[65]

(iii) Ms-SNuPE

Ms-SNuPE is a variation of SNuPE, or Single-Nucleotide Primer Extension, which interrogates the nucleotide present at a selected position to genotype single-nucleotide polymorphisms.[66] In the SNuPE method, the DNA region is amplified by PCR, then annealed to a primer that terminates one base short of the position of interest. The single base incorporated into that position can then be identified by using either radioactively or fluorescently labelled nucleotides. In Ms-SNuPE, the same approach is followed, but the DNA is first bisulfite treated so that differences in sequence are not due to allelic variation but due to methylation status.[67] Ms-SNuPE has been combined with HeavyMethyl PCR to detect colorectal cancer–specific methylation in cirDNA.[68]

Illumina Methylation Arrays

Illumina methylation arrays interrogate the methylation status of selected individual CpG sites. Unlike the PCR-based methods described previously, the methylation arrays are considered a "whole genome" analysis approach. Early versions of the arrays targeted around 27,000 individual CpG sites (27K Array), mostly positioned within promoter CpG islands. The throughput was then increased to approximately 450,000 CpG sites and most recently, 850,000 CpG sites (HM450K Array and MethylationEPIC BeadChip, respectively). The EPIC array has broader coverage and includes a greater range of genomic elements in which methylation is known to play a regulatory role.[69] The array method is based on the Infinium genotyping assay but interrogates differences at CpG sites, rather than single-nucleotide polymorphisms.[70] Bisulfite conversion and whole genome amplification of DNA are followed by binding to bead-coded complementary DNA probes, which stop one base short of the residue of interest. A polymerase then extends the bead bound probe by a single residue, which can be identified by fluorescent labelling, thus revealing the methylation state of the CpG site.

Along with technical developments that increase the number of methylation sites analyzed, there has been a progressive reduction in the amount of input DNA required, with the MethylationEPIC BeadChip specifying 250 ng input DNA. Moss and colleagues were able to reach the 250 ng input requirement by using large blood draws (20 mL) and pooling cirDNA from multiple donors. This allowed them to characterize genome-wide methylation in cirDNA and identify the dominant tissue(s) that contribute to the cirDNA pool in healthy individuals.[8]

Bisulfite Sequencing of CirDNA

Analysis of cirDNA methylation following bisulfite treatment can also be identified directly by next-generation sequencing. Sequencing can analyze either the whole genome or targeted regions of interest. As with other methods in cirDNA research, the challenge in applying this approach is that sequencing protocols typically require DNA input quantities that are not easily obtained from biological samples, with whole genome bisulfite sequencing (WGBS) generally requiring more input DNA. WGBS of cirDNA has been successfully applied; for example, Jensen and colleagues applied WGBS to cirDNA from pregnant women to study the DNA fraction derived from the placenta,[71] while Sun and colleagues used it to identify the tissues that contribute to the cirDNA pool in pregnant women, and in patients with liver cancer and follicular lymphoma.[11] Other studies using next-generation sequencing of bisulfite-treated DNA have used a target approach; Lehmann-Werman and colleagues used targeted parallel sequencing of three hepatocyte markers to observe the increase in liver-derived cirDNA in patients following liver transplantation and patients with sepsis.[13] Similarly, Lam *et al.* reported next-generation sequencing of targeted panels to detect DNA methylation in cirDNA.[26]

Bisulfite-Free Methods for CirDNA Methylation Evaluation

Although the majority of published studies of cirDNA methylation rely on methods incorporating a bisulfite conversion step, bisulfite-free methods have also been applied. These methods have the advantage that the degradation of DNA resulting from bisulfite treatment is avoided; however, they do generally require higher DNA inputs than the commonly used methylation-specific PCR following bisulfite treatment. Nonetheless, they provide an alternative approach.

Methylation-Sensitive Restriction Enzyme Digest

One bisulfite-free approach is to restrict the DNA included in the analysis to the methylated target sequence by removing the unmethylated sequence with a methylation-sensitive restriction enzyme (MSRE). For example, HpaII and Hin6I only cut unmethylated DNA, effectively removing it from the sample. The remaining methylated target can then be quantitated by standard qPCR or analyzed by other methods. As mentioned previously, the sample does not undergo the additional fragmentation and DNA loss associated with bisulfite treatment; however, targets are limited to those DNA regions that contain the appropriate restriction site. This type of technique has been applied to colorectal cancer,[72] breast cancer,[73] and lymphoma.[74]

The MethDet56 assay is based on enrichment of the methylated target by MSRE digest, followed by PCR amplification and microarray quantification.[75] Variations on the method employing methylation capture rather than MSRE, and readouts other than microarray have also been proposed.[75] The assay works on as little as 200 pg of input DNA, making it well suited to cirDNA analyses[75]; however, as with other MSRE-based techniques, it is limited by the locations of restriction enzyme sites. The MethDet56 assay has been applied to measuring pre- and post-treatment cirDNA changes in ER-positive breast cancer patients,[76] differentiating between pancreatitis and pancreatic cancer[77] and between benign and malignant ovarian tumors.[78] One weakness of the MethDet56 assay is that with 56 methylation targets, large numbers of patient samples are needed to achieve statistical significance after correction for multiple comparisons. However, this can be addressed by follow-up studies once a more limited set of candidate biomarkers has been identified by the initial exploratory analysis.

Methylation Capture and Sequencing

Selective capture of methylated DNA followed by sequencing can identify the methylated DNA regions in samples. This approach has been widely applied to tissues but has been more challenging in cirDNA samples due to the high DNA inputs required. Shen and colleagues successfully carried out cell-free methylated DNA precipitation and high-throughput sequencing (cfMeDIP-seq) to identify methylated cirDNA regions in cancer patient plasma and infer the site tumor origin.[79] A key step in developing the protocol was optimizing the method for low DNA inputs. In control experiments, the authors were able to use as little as 1–10 ng of sheared input DNA and recapitulate results obtained from standard Me-DIP, reduced representation bisulfite sequencing (RRBS), and WGBS, which require 100 ng, 1000 ng, and 2000 ng of DNA, respectively.

A methylation capture-and-sequence approach based on methyl-binding protein (MethylMiner, Invitrogen) has been applied to cirDNA, but, once again, the standard protocol used for genomic DNA from tissue was adjusted to accommodate the low inputs of available cirDNA.[29] Specifically, the protocol was scaled down to limit nonspecific binding to excess bead surface area, and the stringency of the wash steps was increased. Successful next-generation sequencing was carried out using only 50 ng of cirDNA input per sample, with the low DNA input mitigated by avoiding the loss of sample that occurs at the gel purification size restriction step, which has been estimated to be up to 95%.[80] Clonal sequencing was used to confirm that the method was specific in identifying methylated and unmethylated DNA regions.[29]

Tissue Selection to Identify Methylated cirDNA Cancer Biomarkers

Cancer-related DNA methylation changes can be identified by comparing tumor methylation with adjacent normal tissue. Since the quantity of DNA obtained from tissues is generally high, laboratory techniques for biomarker discovery in tissue are not limited by the amount of available input material. However, for the purpose of methylated cirDNA biomarker discovery, the DNA methylation of the healthy tissue-of-origin is not relevant if that tissue does not contribute to the cirDNA pool in healthy individuals. For example, *14-3-3 sigma* is methylated in 96% of breast cancers, and unmethylated in healthy breast epithelium; however, it cannot be used as a ctDNA biomarker because it is also methylated in leukocytes.[18]

The appropriate negative controls for excluding DNA methylation present in cirDNA from healthy individuals are tissues that normally contribute to cirDNA, but, until recently, it wasn't known what those tissues were. Leukocytes were the obvious candidate for a major cirDNA contributor, and experimentally this has shown to be the case.[47] However, erythrocyte progenitors,[8,47] endothelial cells,[8] and, less obviously, hepatocytes,[8,11,13] also contribute significant amounts, with erythrocyte progenitors and endothelial cells together accounting for around 40% of the total.[8] This is an example of how a good understanding of cirDNA biology in healthy individuals can inform and advance biomarker discovery. Further work is required to characterize how the cirDNA pool changes in various healthy physiological states (e.g., following exercise and during menstruation), and during common minor illnesses (e.g., respiratory tract infection), if a high specificity of cancer biomarkers is to be achieved from tissue-based discovery strategies.

One benefit of not using the healthy counterpart of the tumor tissue to exclude biomarkers is that it allows inclusion of regions that are methylated in the healthy tissue but don't normally appear in the cirDNA pool. In that scenario, the biomarker would not be indicative of a cancer-associated methylation pattern, but rather, of a particular tissue experiencing abnormal cell death and turn over, suggestive of carcinogenesis.

Tissue-based discovery strategies generally allow access to large amounts of DNA that lend themselves to genome-wide analyses.[81] Promising biomarker candidates identified in tissue can then be evaluated in plasma samples by methylation-specific PCR, which can test a smaller number of candidates with much greater sensitivity. However, with genome-wide methods being refined to accommodate ever-smaller amounts of input DNA, biomarker discovery directly from plasma is also feasible.[79] The advantage of this strategy is that tissues contributing to the cirDNA pool in healthy control subjects do not need to be separately accounted for and analyzed.

Conclusions

Analysis of cirDNA methylation can generate information about disease states as diverse as cancer, cardiac infarction, and diabetes. A colorectal cancer diagnostic test based on circDNA methylation is already FDA approved and available to patients, and a test for diagnosing and monitoring other cancers are in the development pipeline. As in other areas of cirDNA research, there are gains in sensitivity and specificity to be made from improved analysis techniques, which will in turn lead to more effective clinical applications.

References

1. Bestor TH. (1988) Cloning of a mammalian DNA methyltransferase. *Gene* **74**: 9–12.
2. Greenberg MVC, Bourc'his D. (2019) The diverse roles of DNA methylation in mammalian development and disease. *Nat Rev Mol Cell Biol* **20**: 590–607.
3. Saxonov S, Berg P, Brutlag DL. (2006) A genome-wide analysis of CpG dinucleotides in the human genome distinguishes two distinct classes of promoters. *Proc Natl Acad Sci U S A* **103**: 1412–1417. doi:10.073/pnas.0510310103. Epub 2006 Jan 23.
4. Bergman Y, Cedar H. (2013) DNA methylation dynamics in health and disease. *Nat Struct Mol Biol* **20**: 274–281. doi: 10.1038/nsmb.2518.
5. Dor Y, Cedar H. (2018) Principles of DNA methylation and their implications for biology and medicine. *Lancet* **392**: 777–786. doi:10.1016/S0140-6736(18)31268-6. Epub 2018 Aug 9.
6. Jones PA. (2012) Functions of DNA methylation: Islands, start sites, gene bodies and beyond. *Nat Rev Genet* **13**: 484–492. doi:10.1038/nrg3230.
7. Schubeler D. (2015) Function and information content of DNA methylation. *Nature* **517**: 321–326. doi:10.1038/nature14192.
8. Moss J, Magenheim J, Neiman D, *et al.* (2018) Comprehensive human cell-type methylation atlas reveals origins of circulating cell-free DNA in health and disease. *Nat Commun* **9**: 5068. doi:10.1038/s41467-018-07466-6.
9. Guo S, Diep D, Plongthongkum N, Fung HL, Zhang K, Zhang K. (2017) Identification of methylation haplotype blocks aids in deconvolution of heterogeneous tissue samples and tumor tissue-of-origin mapping from plasma DNA. *Nat Genet* **49**: 635–642. doi:10.1038/ng.3805. Epub 2017 Mar 6.
10. Lam WKJ, Gai W, Sun K, *et al.* (2017) DNA of erythroid origin is present in human plasma and informs the types of Anemia. *Clin Chem* **63**: 1614–1623. doi:10.373/clinchem.2017.272401. Epub 2017 Aug 7.

11. Sun K, Jiang P, Chan KC, *et al.* (2015) Plasma DNA tissue mapping by genome-wide methylation sequencing for noninvasive prenatal, cancer, and transplantation assessments. *Proc Natl Acad Sci U S A* **112**: E5503–E5512. doi: 10.1073/pnas.1508736112. Epub 2015 Sep 21.

12. Lehmann-Werman R, Neiman D, Zemmour H, *et al.* (2016) Identification of tissue-specific cell death using methylation patterns of circulating DNA. *Proc Natl Acad Sci U S A* **113**: E1826–34. doi: 10.073/pnas.1519286113. Epub 2016 Mar 14.

13. Lehmann-Werman R, Magenheim J, Moss J, *et al.* (2018). Monitoring liver damage using hepatocyte-specific methylation markers in cell-free circulating DNA. *JCI Insight* **3**: 120687. doi:10.1172/jci.insight

14. Jones PA, Baylin SB. (2007) The epigenomics of cancer. *Cell* **128**: 683–692. doi:10.1016/j.cell.2007.01.029.

15. Clark SJ, Melki J. (2002) DNA methylation and gene silencing in cancer: Which is the guilty party? *Oncogene* **21**: 5380–5387.

16. Lee ST, Wiemels JL. (2016) Genome-wide CpG island methylation and intergenic demethylation propensities vary among different tumor sites. *Nucleic Acids Res* **44**: 1105–1117. doi: 10.093/nar/gkv038. Epub 2015 Oct 12.

17. Montavon C, Gloss BS, Warton K, *et al.* (2012) Prognostic and diagnostic significance of DNA methylation patterns in high grade serous ovarian cancer. *Gynecol Oncol* **124**: 582–588.

18. Umbricht CB, Evron E, Gabrielson E, Ferguson A, Marks J, Sukumar S. (2001) Hypermethylation of 14-3-3 sigma (stratifin) is an early event in breast cancer. *Oncogene* **20**: 3348–3353.

19. Locke WJ, Guanzon D, Ma C, *et al.* (2019) DNA methylation cancer biomarkers: Translation to the clinic. *Front Genet* **10**: 1150.

20. Vogelstein B, Papadopoulos N, Velculescu VE, Zhou S, Diaz LA, Jr., Kinzler KW. (2013) Cancer genome landscapes. *Science* **339**: 1546–1558.

21. Network TCGA. (2012) Comprehensive molecular portraits of human breast tumours. *Nature* **490**: 61–70. doi: 10.1038/nature11412. Epub 2012 Sep 23.

22. Ahmed AA, Etemadmoghadam D, Temple J, *et al.* (2010) Driver mutations in TP53 are ubiquitous in high grade serous carcinoma of the ovary. *J Pathol* **221**: 49–56. doi: 10.1002/path.2696.

23. Kandoth C, Schultz N, Cherniack AD, *et al.* (2013) Integrated genomic characterization of endometrial carcinoma. *Nature* **497**: 67–73. doi: 10.1038/nature12113.

24. Diehl F, Schmidt K, Choti MA, *et al.* (2008) Circulating mutant DNA to assess tumor dynamics. *Nat Med* **14**: 985–990.

25. Forshew T, Murtaza M, Parkinson C, *et al.* (2012) Noninvasive identification and monitoring of cancer mutations by targeted deep sequencing of plasma DNA. *Sci Transl Med.* **4**: 136ra68. doi: 10.1126/scitranslmed.3003726.

26. Lam D, Luu PL, Song JZ, *et al.* (2020) Comprehensive evaluation of targeted multiplex bisulphite PCR sequencing for validation of DNA methylation biomarker panels. *Clin Epigenetics* **12**: 90.

27. Li Y, Tollefsbol TO. (2011) DNA methylation detection: Bisulfite genomic sequencing analysis. *Methods Mol Biol* **791**: 11–21.

28. Feng S, Zhong Z, Wang M, Jacobsen SE. (2020) Efficient and accurate determination of genome-wide DNA methylation patterns in Arabidopsis thaliana with enzymatic methyl sequencing. *Epigenetics Chromatin* **13**: 42.

29. Warton K, Lin V, Navin T, *et al.* (2014) Methylation-capture and next-generation sequencing of free circulating DNA from human plasma. *BMC Genomics* **15**: 476. doi: 10.1186/471-2164-15-476

30. Nair SS, Coolen MW, Stirzaker C, *et al.* (2011) Comparison of methyl-DNA immunoprecipitation (MeDIP) and methyl-CpG binding domain (MBD) protein capture for genome-wide DNA methylation analysis reveal CpG sequence coverage bias. *Epigenetics* **6**: 34–44.

31. Frommer M, McDonald LE, Millar DS, *et al.* (1992) A genomic sequencing protocol that yields a positive display of 5-methylcytosine residues in individual DNA strands. *Proc Natl Acad Sci U S A* **89**: 1827–1831.

32. Clark SJ, Harrison J, Paul CL, Frommer M. (1994) High sensitivity mapping of methylated cytosines. *Nucleic Acids Res* **22**: 2990–2997.

33. Clark S, Frommer M. (1995) Deamination with NaHSO3 in DNA methylation studies in: DNA and nucleoprotein structure in vivo. *Biomedical Publishers*. RG Landes Company, Austin & Springer-Verlag, New York, pp. 123–132.

34. Holmes EE, Jung M, Meller S, *et al.* (2014) Performance evaluation of kits for bisulfite-conversion of DNA from tissues, cell lines, FFPE tissues, aspirates, lavages, effusions, plasma, serum, and urine. *PLOS ONE* **9**: e93933. doi: 10.1371/journal.pone.0093933. eCollection 2014.

35. Leontiou CA, Hadjidaniel MD, Mina P, Antoniou P, Ioannides M, Patsalis PC. (2015) Bisulfite conversion of DNA: Performance comparison of different kits and methylation quantitation of epigenetic biomarkers that have the potential to be used in non-invasive prenatal testing. *PLOS ONE* **10**: e0135058. doi: 10.1371/journal.pone.0135058.

36. Worm Orntoft MB, Jensen SO, Hansen TB, Bramsen JB, Andersen CL. (2017) Comparative analysis of 12 different kits for bisulfite conversion of circulating cell-free DNA. *Epigenetics* **12**: 626–636. doi: 10.1080/15592294.2017.1334024. Epub 2017 May 30.

37. Yi S, Long F, Cheng J, Huang D. (2017) An optimized rapid bisulfite conversion method with high recovery of cell-free DNA. *BMC Mol Biol* **18**: 24. doi: 10.1186/s12867-017-0101-4.

38. Werner B, Yuwono NL, Henry C, *et al.* (2019) Circulating cell-free DNA from plasma undergoes less fragmentation during bisulfite treatment than genomic DNA due to low molecular weight. *PLOS ONE* **14**: e0224338. doi: 10.1371/journal.pone.. eCollection 2019.

39. Millar DS, Warnecke PM, Melki JR, Clark SJ. (2002) Methylation sequencing from limiting DNA: Embryonic, fixed, and microdissected cells. *Methods* **27**: 108–113.

40. Millar D, Christova Y, Holliger P. (2015) A polymerase engineered for bisulfite sequencing. *Nucleic Acids Res* **43**: e155. doi: 10.1093/nar/gkv798. Epub 2015 Aug 13.

41. Warnecke PM, Stirzaker C, Song J, Grunau C, Melki JR, Clark SJ. (2002) Identification and resolution of artifacts in bisulfite sequencing. *Methods* **27**: 101–107.

42. Church TR, Wandell M, Lofton-Day C, *et al.* (2002) Prospective evaluation of methylated SEPT9 in plasma for detection of asymptomatic colorectal cancer. *Gut* **63**: 317–325. doi: 10.1136/gutjnl-2012-304149. Epub 2013 Feb 13.

43. Andersen RF, Spindler KL, Brandslund I, Jakobsen A, Pallisgaard N. (2015) Improved sensitivity of circulating tumor DNA measurement using short PCR amplicons. *Clin Chim Acta* **439**: 97–101.

44. Grunau C, Clark SJ, Rosenthal A. (2001) Bisulfite genomic sequencing: Systematic investigation of critical experimental parameters. *Nucleic Acids Res* **29**: E65–E5.

45. Jones PA, Baylin SB. (2002) The fundamental role of epigenetic events in cancer. *Nat Rev Genet* **3**: 415–428.

46. Snyder MW, Kircher M, Hill AJ, Daza RM, Shendure J. (2016) Cell-free DNA comprises an in vivo nucleosome footprint that informs its tissues-of-origin. *Cell* **164**: 57–68.

47. Jahr S, Hentze H, Englisch S, *et al.* (2001) DNA fragments in the blood plasma of cancer patients: Quantitations and evidence for their origin from apoptotic and necrotic cells. *Cancer Res* **61**: 1659–1665.

48. Smith GM, Whelan J, Pescini R, Ghersa P, DeLamarter JF, Hooft van Huijsduijnen R. (1993) DNA-methylation of the E-selectin promoter represses NF-kappa B transactivation. *Biochem Biophys Res Commun* **194**: 215–221.

49. Stadhouders R, Pas SD, Anber J, Voermans J, Mes TH, Schutten M. (2010) The effect of primer-template mismatches on the detection and quantification of nucleic acids using the 5′ nuclease assay. *J Mol Diagn* **12**: 109–117.

50. Ghedira R, Papazova N, Vuylsteke M, Ruttink T, Taverniers I, De Loose M. (2009) Assessment of primer/template mismatch effects on real-time PCR amplification of target taxa for GMO quantification. *J Agric Food Chem* **57**: 9370–9377. doi: 10.1021/jf901976a.

51. Warnecke PM, Stirzaker C, Melki JR, Millar DS, Paul CL, Clark SJ. (1997) Detection and measurement of PCR bias in quantitative methylation analysis of bisulphite-treated DNA. *Nucleic Acids Res* **25**: 4422–4426.

52. Clark SJ, Statham A, Stirzaker C, Molloy PL, Frommer M. (2006) DNA methylation: Bisulphite modification and analysis. *Nat Protoc* **1**: 2353–2364.

53. Strien J, Sanft J, Mall G. (2013) Enhancement of PCR amplification of moderate GC-containing and highly GC-rich DNA sequences. *Mol Biotechnol* **54**: 1048–1054.

54. Philipp AB, Nagel D, Stieber P, *et al.* (2014) Circulating cell-free methylated DNA and lactate dehydrogenase release in colorectal cancer. *BMC Cancer* **14**: 245. doi: 10.1186/471-2407-14-245.

55. Matuschek C, Bolke E, Lammering G, *et al.* (2010) Methylated APC and GSTP1 genes in serum DNA correlate with the presence of circulating blood tumor cells and are associated with a more aggressive and advanced breast cancer disease. *Eur J Med Res* **15**: 277–286.

56. Rand K, Qu W, Ho T, Clark SJ, Molloy P. (2002) Conversion-specific detection of DNA methylation using real-time polymerase chain reaction (ConLight-MSP) to avoid false positives. *Methods* **27**: 114–120.

57. Quan PL, Sauzade M, Brouzes E. (2018) dPCR: A technology review. *Sensors (Basel)* **18**: 1271.

58. Li M, Chen WD, Papadopoulos N, *et al.* (2009) Sensitive digital quantification of DNA methylation in clinical samples. *Nat Biotechnol* **27**: 858–863. doi: 10.1038/nbt.559

59. Barault L, Amatu A, Bleeker FE, *et al.* (2015) Digital PCR quantification of MGMT methylation refines prediction of clinical benefit from alkylating agents in glioblastoma and metastatic colorectal cancer. *Ann Oncol* **26**: 1994–1999. doi: 10.093/annonc/mdv272. Epub 2015 Jun 25.

60. Overman MJ, Morris V, Moinova H, *et al.* (2016) Phase I/II study of azacitidine and capecitabine/oxaliplatin (CAPOX) in refractory CIMP-high metastatic colorectal cancer: Evaluation of circulating methylated vimentin. *Oncotarget* **7**: 67495–67506. doi: 10.18632/oncotarget.1317.

61. Rand KN, Ho T, Qu W, *et al.* (2005) Headloop suppression PCR and its application to selective amplification of methylated DNA sequences. *Nucleic Acids Res* **33**: e127. doi: 10.1093/nar/gni120.

62. Mahon KL, Qu W, Devaney J, *et al.* (2014) Methylated glutathione S-transferase 1 (mGSTP1) is a potential plasma free DNA epigenetic marker of prognosis and response to chemotherapy in castrate-resistant prostate cancer. *Br J Cancer* **111**: 1802–1809. doi: 10.038/bjc.2014.463. Epub Aug 21.

63. Mahon KL, Qu W, Lin HM, *et al.* (2018) Serum free methylated glutathione S-transferase 1 DNA levels, survival, and response to docetaxel in metastatic, castration-resistant prostate cancer: Post hoc analyses of data from a phase 3 trial. *Eur Urol* **19**: 30855–30858.

64. Cottrell SE, Distler J, Goodman NS, *et al.* (2004) A real-time PCR assay for DNA-methylation using methylation-specific blockers. *Nucleic Acids Res* **32**: e10. doi: 1093/nar/gnh008.

65. Lofton-Day C, Model F, Devos T, *et al.* (2008) DNA methylation biomarkers for blood-based colorectal cancer screening. *Clin Chem* **54**: 414–423. doi: 10.1373/clinchem.2007.095992. Epub 2007 Dec 18.

66. Greenwood AD, Burke DT. (1996) Single nucleotide primer extension: Quantitative range, variability, and multiplex analysis. *Genome Res* **6**: 336–348.

67. Gonzalgo ML, Liang G. (2007) Methylation-sensitive single-nucleotide primer extension (Ms-SNuPE) for quantitative measurement of DNA methylation. *Nat Protoc* **2**: 1931–1936. doi: 10.038/nprot.2007.271.

68. Tierling S, Schuster M, Tetzner R, Walter J. (2010) A combined HM-PCR/SNuPE method for high sensitive detection of rare DNA methylation. *Epigenetics Chromatin* **3**: 12. doi: 0.1186/756-8935-3-12.

69. Pidsley R, Zotenko E, Peters TJ, *et al.* (2016) Critical evaluation of the illumina MethylationEPIC BeadChip microarray for whole-genome DNA methylation profiling. *Genome Biol* **17**: 208.

70. Bibikova M, Barnes B, Tsan C, *et al.* (2011) High density DNA methylation array with single CpG site resolution. *Genomics* **98**: 288–295. doi: 10.1016/j.ygeno.2011.07.007. Epub Aug 2.

71. Jensen TJ, Kim SK, Zhu Z, *et al.* (2015) Whole genome bisulfite sequencing of cell-free DNA and its cellular contributors uncovers placenta hypomethylated domains. *Genome Biol* **16**: 78. doi: 10.1186/s13059-015-0645-x.

72. Bhangu JS, Beer A, Mittlbock M, *et al.* (2018) Circulating free methylated tumor DNA markers for sensitive assessment of tumor burden and early response monitoring in patients receiving systemic chemotherapy for colorectal cancer liver metastasis. *Ann Surg* **268**: 894–902. doi: 10.1097/SLA.0000000000002901.

73. Kristiansen S, Nielsen D, Soletormos G. (2016) Detection and monitoring of hypermethylated RASSF1A in serum from patients with metastatic breast cancer. **8**: 35. doi:10.1186/s13148-016-0199-0. eCollection 2016.

74. Deligezer U, Yaman F, Erten N, Dalay N. (2003) Frequent copresence of methylated DNA and fragmented nucleosomal DNA in plasma of lymphoma patients. *Clin Chim Acta* **335**: 89–94.

75. Levenson VV, Melnikov AA. (2011) The MethDet: A technology for biomarker development. *Expert Rev Mol Diagn* **11**: 807–812. doi: 10.1586/erm.11.74

76. Liggett TE, Melnikov AA, Marks JR, Levenson VV. (2011) Methylation patterns in cell-free plasma DNA reflect removal of the primary tumor and drug treatment of breast cancer patients. *Int J Cancer* **128**: 492–499. doi: 10.1002/ijc.25363. Epub 2010 Apr 5.

77. Liggett T, Melnikov A, Yi QL, *et al.* (2010) Differential methylation of cell-free circulating DNA among patients with pancreatic cancer versus chronic pancreatitis. *Cancer* **116**: 1674–1680. doi: 10.002/cncr.24893.

78. Liggett TE, Melnikov A, Yi Q, *et al.* (2011) Distinctive DNA methylation patterns of cell-free plasma DNA in women with malignant ovarian tumors.

Gynecol Oncol **120**: 113–120. doi: 10.1016/j.ygyno.2010.09.019. Epub Nov 6.

79. Shen SY, Singhania R, Fehringer G, *et al.* (2018) Sensitive tumour detection and classification using plasma cell-free DNA methylomes. *Nature* **563**: 579–583. doi: 10.1038/s41586-018-0703-0. Epub 2018 Nov 14.

80. Quail MA, Kozarewa I, Smith F, *et al.* (2008) A large genome center's improvements to the Illumina sequencing system. *Nat Methods* **5**: 1005–1010. doi: 10.38/nmeth.270.

81. Charlton J, Williams RD, Weeks M, *et al.* (2014) Methylome analysis identifies a Wilms tumor epigenetic biomarker detectable in blood. *Genome Biol* **15**: 434. doi: 10.1186/s13059-014-0434-y.

Index

apoptosis, 10, 27, 114, 119, 140,
141, 176, 178–182, 185–188,
198, 248
apoptotic bodies, 211, 223
assays to monitor the DNase
activity, 189

biobanking, 22, 29, 36, 47–55, 59,
64, 65, 105
biomarker discovery, 53, 54, 268,
269
biospecimens, 24, 31, 37, 47–54,
58
bisulfite conversion of DNA,
30, 58, 64, 96, 97,123, 124,
250–258, 261, 263–267
blood-derived PCR inhibitors,
52, 53, 58, 59 88, 127
blood DNAses, 24, 27, 175–199
blood storage and handling,
21–41, 47–55, 185, 198, 225, 253
broad consent, 50

capturing shorter DNA
fragments, 10, 78, 79, 88, 92,
93, 95, 104, 115, 117, 126,
144–146, 160, 252, 254
cell autonomous nucleases, 185
cell-free methylated DNA
precipitation and high-
throughput sequencing
(cfMeDIP-seq), 267
cell nonautonomous nucleases,
185
cell-of-origin biomarker, 4, 96,
113, 114, 120, 217, 248, 255,
267, 268
cirDNA cleavage signature, 116,
141, 175, 180, 181
cirDNA library, 4, 10, 12, 92, 115,
117, 139–154, 159–161, 220,
221
cirDNA methylation, 3, 22, 27,
30, 58, 65, 34, 35, 97, 98,
116–118, 120, 122–124,
247–270
cirDNA methylation as a cancer
biomarker, 3, 22, 34, 117,
118, 249, 250, 254, 262, 263,
266–269

cirDNA origin, 10, 27, 114, 119, 140, 141, 176, 178–182, 185–188, 198, 248

cirDNA storage, 30, 48, 51, 55,

cirDNA yield, 6, 10, 11, 23–25, 27–28, 40, 55, 58, 63–106, 150, 176, 196, 253

clinical data management, 49–51

clonal evolution, 3, 153

column-based cirDNA purification, 63, 66–68, 77, 79, 84, 88

concentration of cirDNA in plasma, 5–7, 29, 54–57, 66, 88–90, 94, 96, 100, 140, 143, 163, 185, 186, 191, 250

CpG dinucleotide, 123, 125, 247, 248, 256, 259, 260, 264

CpG islands, 125, 248, 249, 254, 264

degradation of DNA, 9–11, 13, 27, 30, 50, 176, 179, 180, 184, 190, 196

density gradient isolation techniques, 211, 226–228, 232, 233, 235

detecting disease recurrence, 3, 21, 49, 118, 164, 212

dexosomes, 210

digital PCR (dPCR), 6, 10, 28, 37, 38, 40, 41, 64, 121–124, 122, 131, 141–143, 158, 233, 259, 261

DNA degradation, 9–11, 13, 27, 30, 50, 176, 179, 180, 184, 190, 196

DNA methylation, 22, 27, 30, 58, 96, 97, 116–118, 120, 123, 125, 247–270

DNA Protection by Nucleosome Structure, 36, 56, 66, 96, 114, 115, 116, 120, 125, 126, 180–182, 186, 187, 254, 255

double-stranded DNA library preparation, 144, 145, 150

early detection and diagnosis of cancer, 3, 7, 49, 52, 53, 157

enrichment of ctDNA, 4, 11–13, 84, 87, 146, 150, 156, 213

enzymatic cytosine conversion, 250

ethical considerations, 50, 51

exosomal biogenesis, 210, 214–216

exosomal cargo, 210–212, 216–219

exosomal fingerprint, 212, 217

exosomal isolation strategies, 224

exosomal loading, 212

experimental artifacts, 5, 55, 56, 126, 175, 197, 198, 221, 233, 234, 255,

field flow fractionation (FFF), 231

fluorescent dyes, 55, 121, 128, 129, 142, 189–192, 230, 258,

formalin-fixed paraffin embedded (FFPE), 13, 253

headloop suppression PCR, 262

healthy controls, 22, 48, 53, 83, 86, 90–92, 94, 125, 128, 141, 184, 188, 268, 269

HeavyMethyl, 263
hematopoietic cell death, 114,
178
hemolysis, 37, 224
hemolytic index, 37

Illumina methylation arrays, 255,
264
Illumina platforms, 97, 142, 255,
254
intercellular communication,
210–212

library preparation kits, 115, 144,
220
lipid bilayer membranes, 209,
212, 219, 225
liquid-liquid cirDNA purification,
66, 74, 80–82, 84, 88, 91
low-abundance in plasma/serum,
6, 63–65, 98, 104, 106, 252

magnetic bead, 57, 63, 68, 79, 80,
87, 89, 94, 97, 100
matrix binding, 63, 66–68, 77, 79,
82, 84, 88, 230, 261
methylation-sensitive restriction
enzyme (MSRE), 266
methylation-specific PCR, 249,
255, 256, 260
methylation-specific primers,
255, 260
methylation unbiased PCR, 256
Methyl-BEAMing (Beads
Emulsion Amplification
Magnetics), 261

microfluidic DNA gel
electrophoresis, 38, 64, 69,
71–73, 89, 105, 142
microvesicles, 211
minimal residual disease
detection, 3, 118
mitochondrial DNA, 65, 92, 93,
116, 117, 120
monitoring of cancer, 3, 57, 64,
106, 118, 139, 155, 156, 164,
212, 263, 269
Ms-SNuPE, 263

nanoparticle tracking analysis,
222
nanovesicles, 210
Next-generation sequencing
(NGS), 6, 57, 92, 139–164
NGS library preparation
protocols, 115, 139–164, 265,
267
noninvasive tumor genotyping,
3
nucleases, 4, 9, 11, 12, 114, 116,
117, 141, 175–199
nucleosome positioning, 36, 56,
66, 96, 114, 115, 116, 120, 125,
126, 180–182, 186, 187, 254,
255

optimal volume of plasma, 53

phenol–chloroform protocols, 63,
69, 74, 76, 81–85, 97, 100
polyethylene glycol (PEG)
precipitation, 228

preanalytical handling, 5, 10,
21–41, 50, 64, 79, 105, 175,
191, 196, 197, 224
predicting and/or monitoring
response to therapy, 8, 49, 64,
212
primer binding, 124, 125, 129,
158, 163, 263
primer/probe design, 113, 129,
254, 259
processing of blood specimens, 5,
10, 22, 23, 29, 33, 50, 55, 193,
198, 224, 225, 253
protein surfaceome, 213

QIAamp Circulating Nucleic
Acid kit, 63, 68, 71–74, 76–80,
82, 84, 86–93, 95–97, 99,
101–105

quality assurance, 31

recurrence monitoring, 3, 57, 64,
106, 118, 139, 155, 156, 164,
212, 263, 269
reporting results, 51

sequencing-based methods,
139–164
sequencing library preparation,
113, 139–164
single-stranded library
preparation, 115, 117, 145, 146
size exclusion chromatography
(SEC), 229
SNuPE, or Single-Nucleotide
Primer Extension, 263
standardized operating
procedures (SOPs) for
specimen collection and
processing, 49

transmission electron microscopy
(TEM), 221
treatment monitoring, 3, 49, 57,
64, 118, 139, 156, 164, 212,
263, 269

ultracentrifugation, 211, 226

ultrafiltration, 228
unique molecular identifiers
(UMIs), 147